The information in this book has been carefully reviewed by experienced clinicians in this field and is based on the best data currently available.

If a specific ingredient or over-the-counter product that you are looking for is not included in this book, please contact Dr. Nice through www.DrNiceProducts.com.

The BREASTFEEDING *Family's Guide to* NONPRESCRIPTION DRUGS *and* EVERYDAY PRODUCTS

By Frank J. Nice, RPh, DPA, CPHP

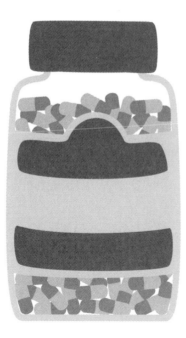

Platypus Media, LLC
Washington, D.C.

The author does not warrant the safety of the medications included in this book, but only reviews the current state of knowledge in this field. Ultimately, the use of these medications in combination with breastfeeding must be reviewed by a knowledgeable clinician, together with the breastfeeding parent, to evaluate the relative safety of any particular product. No medical or legal responsibility is assumed by the author or publisher.

The Breastfeeding Family's Guide to Nonprescription Drugs and Everyday Products
Written by Frank J. Nice, RPh, DPA, CPHP

Text © 2023 Frank J. Nice
Cover art © 2023 Platypus Media, LLC

Editing, Design, and Cover by Hannah Thelen
Copyeditors: Caitlin Burnham, Marlee Brooks

Paperback ISBN 13: 978-1-951995-10-2
  First Edition • May 2023
eBook ISBN 13: 978-1-951995-11-9
  First Edition • May 2023

Published in the United States by:
  Platypus Media, LLC
  750 First Street NE, Suite 700
  Washington, DC 20002
  202-546-1674 • Fax: 202-558-2132
  www.PlatypusMedia.com • Info@PlatypusMedia.com

Distributed to the book trade by:
  National Book Network (North America)
    301-459-3366 • Toll-free: 800-462-6420
    CustomerCare@NBNbooks.com • NBNbooks.com
  NBN international (worldwide)
    NBNi.Cservs@IngramContent.com • Distribution.NBNi.co.uk

Library of Congress Control Number: 2023931001

10 9 8 7 6 5 4 3 2 1

Dedication

As always, to my wife, Myung Hee, who has graciously supported me over my many years of breastfeeding counseling, and innumerable hours spent hovering over my laptop to produce my books.

Forever, to my Polish grandparents and parents who sacrificed much to allow me to practice as a pharmacist.

To all the numerous lactation consultants, healthcare professionals, friends, and students who have encouraged me over the past 45 years.

To all breastfeeding mothers and children, and especially to those breastfeeding mothers of Haiti whom I have been privileged to serve for the past 25 years. Despite all that you endure, you persevere because breast is best.

Almost last, but not least, I am especially grateful to my editor, Hannah Thelen, who took what I thought was a really good third edition of *Nonprescription Drugs for the Breastfeeding Mother* and turned it into a blockbuster new title.

Finally, to my awesome God, who has made my professional career as a pharmacist a true one-of-a-kind blessing.

~

Acknowledgements

I especially acknowledge my father, Frank Sr., who drove a coal truck, and my grandfathers, Philip and George, who worked deep down in the coal mines. My mother, Irene, and my grandmothers, Sophia and Catherine, all stood by their men as they worked their dangerous trades. Their Polish perseverance ensured that I was the first in my family not only to attend college, but also to become a pharmacist.

Three republic countries have provided the backgrounds for my ability to practice as a pharmacist and to use my God-given skills to hopefully make the world a better place because of what I have been able to do with my life.

I am truly indebted to and thankful to the nations and citizens of the United States, Poland, and Haiti. I am indebted to all my fellow uniformed and military service veterans who served and died to make this all possible. We are and have been truly blessed.

Table of Contents

About the Author

DR. FRANK J. NICE has been an expert consultant, lecturer, and author on medications and breastfeeding for over 45 years. He holds a bachelor's degree in pharmacy, a master's degree in pharmacy administration, master's and doctorate degrees in public administration, and certification in public health pharmacy.

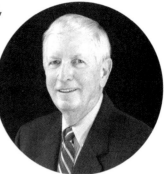

He spent 30 years of distinguished government service with the U.S. Public Health Service. He later practiced at the National Institutes of Health, where he was also an assistant program director of the Clinical Neurosciences Program, before working as a pharmacist and project manager at the Food and Drug Administration. Now retired, he continues to write and lecture in addition to serving as a pharmacy consultant and the president of Dr. Nice's Natural Products.

Dr. Nice has authored over 50 peer-reviewed articles on prescription medications, over-the-counter products, and herbals used during breastfeeding. His books include *Nonprescription Drugs for the Breastfeeding Mother* (the precursor to this book); *The Galactagogue Recipe Book*; and *Recreational Drugs and Drugs Used to Treat Addicted Mothers: Impact on Pregnancy and Breastfeeding*.

Alongside his career as a pharmacist, Dr. Nice has organized and participated in over 60 medical missions to Haiti. He helped start the *Orphelinat Coeur d' Jesus* (Heart of Jesus Orphanage), a K–13 school in Haiti that serves 550 students and houses approximately 50 orphans. He is also a founding member of Health and Education for Haiti (HEH), a nonprofit that aims to address medical, educational, infrastructural, and basic needs for the people of Haiti.

He lives with his wife in the Washington, D.C. metro area. He can be reached through his website: www.DrNiceProducts.com.

Why I Wrote This Book

Beauty can be defined as a quality that gives pleasure or deep satisfaction to the mind, whether arising from sensory manifestations such as shape, color, or sound; a meaningful design or pattern; or something intangible, like a personality, choice, or relationship. That is quite a long definition for the term, yet it still does not do justice to the way we, as humans, experience beauty.

Despite the vagueness of the concept, I think most would agree that there is an undeniable beauty to the concept and art of breastfeeding, the physiology of breasts, and a mother's inherent ability to nourish her child. The Rev. William D. Virtue, in his book, *Mother and Infant: The Moral Theology of Embodied Self-Giving in Motherhood*, exquisitely describes the beauty of breastfeeding: "Maternal breastfeeding is the kind of mothering that fosters formation of the human being in infancy and early childhood." The formation of the human being refers not only to the physical growth of the child, but also to mental, emotional, and spiritual development that can be achieved through nursing.

Human newborns are designed to be breastfed twelve or more times a day. Mother rabbits feed their babies only once a day. Humans are breastfed so often not only because their stomachs are the size of a marble, but also because breastfeeding helps mothers and babies bond almost continuously. Physical touch, an essential part of breastfeeding, is necessary to fulfill a child's need for emotional security and loving attachment. This extensive physical and emotional bonding contributes to well-adjusted adults later on in life. Breastfeeding provides both the perfect food to form the human body, and the perfect means to form the human nature through love, trust, and closeness.

With this in mind, I wanted to create a simple, thorough reference guide to over-the-counter products that are safe to use while breastfeeding. Intended to be used by pharmacists, physicians, nurse practitioners, lactation consultants, midwives, and (of course) parents, it is my hope that this book will help breastfeeding mothers maintain their personal health and minimize any stress, fear, or pain that they may be experiencing. That way, they can focus on what's most important: building a definitively beautiful, lasting bond with their children.

1.

AN IMPORTANT
INTRODUCTION

For Breastfeeding Families

When a breastfeeding mother uses any form of medication, there is a good chance that the ingredients will pass to her infant through her breastmilk. Even if the medication is entirely safe for an adult, there may be harmful consequences for an infant. In fact, there are some very well-known, trusted products that parents should never take while breastfeeding due to the ingredients being unsafe for their breastfed baby. There are also medications that can interfere with breastfeeding by inhibiting breastmilk production.

These problems are easy to avoid when taking a *prescription* medication because doctors will generally understand the circumstances and be able to prescribe something safe. However, the use of a *nonprescription* or *over-the-counter (OTC)* medication does not require professional approval.

Individual consumers usually make their own decisions about using nonprescription medications or other commonly available health and recreation products (such as caffeinated drinks, CBD oil, or melatonin supplements). Most consumers assume that a product for sale in a drugstore or grocery store must be safe to use, but that isn't always the case. Choosing a medication or other product for yourself, especially while breastfeeding, is not as simple as it seems. The labels for OTC products, though vitally important, do not tell you if a medication is safe for breastfeeding. It can be all too easy to unintentionally use something harmful.

Even so, the use of nonprescription or over-the-counter medications by breastfeeding mothers is more common than the use of prescription drugs. The sale and use of these products is a $37 billion industry. Nearly nine out of every ten Americans use OTC medications regularly, which equals over 260 million users. Every year, Americans make approximately three billion trips to purchase OTCs. Because OTCs are available for common and not-so-common maladies, there is an overwhelming and bewildering variety of nonprescription products available to consumers.

To make matters more confusing, nonprescription drugs often consist of multiple ingredients for various symptoms. Many have both regular-strength and extra-strength formulations of the same product. The medication may be short-acting or long-acting. In addition, package directions may be complex or unclear.

For all products, it is best to reference the safety information provided in this book, and consult a pharmacist if there is any doubt. The following basic guidelines can help breastfeeding parents determine which nonprescription medications are safe to use:

- Even when using this book, it is important that your healthcare practitioner assists in evaluating all the possible risks to the breast-feeding parent and infant, particularly when the infant is younger than one month.

- If possible, it is always best to use a non-drug approach to treating your symptoms.

- Avoid taking nonprescription medications for which little breastfeeding information is available. Your pharmacist should be able to assist you in finding this information.

- Always choose the safest products to use while breastfeeding. Once again, your pharmacist can help you determine this.

- Take products with single active ingredients, rather than multiple active ingredients. It is best to take a preparation that has one or two ingredients that will treat a specific condition, rather than exposing the breastfeeding infant to unnecessary ingredients.

- Avoid taking two different products with the same or overlapping active ingredients.

- Take short-acting products rather than long-acting products. This protects the infant from being exposed to a drug for a longer period of time, especially if an adverse reaction is possible.

- Use regular-strength products rather than extra-strength. There is no need for the infant to be exposed to extra amounts of a drug.

- Know the possible side effects that you or your infant might experience. Your pharmacist can help you with this.

- Do not take more than the recommended dose.

- Topical skin preparations applied to sore or cracked nipples should be specifically indicated for this purpose. Even small amounts of medications applied to the nipple can transfer to the infant, so caution is recommended. Generally, if you can see the medication on the nipple, too much has been used.

- Parents of premature infants in particular should always consult with a knowledgeable pharmacist, healthcare provider, or lactation consultant before taking any over-the-counter products.

While this advice may help with decision-making, it's not always clear whether it is safe to use a specific nonprescription medication or product. However, **discontinuing breastfeeding for the purpose of taking a certain medication is not necessary in most instances**. There are very few dangerous medications that do not have a suitable alternative.

The information in this book provides simple, clear answers to help your breastfeeding family choose a safe and effective product for every health need.

For Pharmacists, Lactation Consultants, and Other Healthcare Professionals

Pharmacists play a larger role than any other healthcare professionals in recommending and influencing nonprescription drugs that consumers purchase and use. In most instances, however, whether a consumer is breastfeeding or not is not taken into consideration.

Every year for the past 25 years, *Pharmacy Times* has surveyed pharmacists to see which OTC products are recommended most often. On that list compiled by the journal, there are approximately three dozen OTC products that are unsafe for babies to receive through breastmilk (see page 57 for more information). Included on this unsafe list were products from very well known brands, including Pepto-Bismol, Excedrin, Zicam, and Alka-Seltzer, among others.

There are two critical points to be taken from this observation. Pharmacists, when recommending an OTC product, may not realize that it is going to be used by someone who is breastfeeding. They also may not know if the product is unsafe to use during breastfeeding, particularly when the product or brand is widely recommended or has many variations. Using Zicam as an example, there are some Zicam products that are compatible with breastfeeding, while others are unsafe. This is also true for other OTCs.

As a pharmacist myself, I wrote this book to help healthcare professionals make correct recommendations, and to help consumers ensure that the products they use for themselves are also safe for their infants.

2.
UNDERSTANDING NONPRESCRIPTION DRUGS

How and Why You Should Always Read the Label

It is very important to read the label when using nonprescription drugs, as labeling helps ensure that drugs are used correctly and safely. The Food and Drug Administration (FDA) has issued regulations regarding over-the-counter drug labeling. The regulations enable consumers to choose the best and safest way to use OTC drugs. Using the labeling information in addition to the information provided in this book will maximize the safety and compatibility of selected nonprescription products during breastfeeding.

How is OTC drug labeling different from prescription drugs?

- The label uses common words that are easy to understand.

- The print is larger, making it easier to read.

- The label looks the same for all products and is in the same place on every product.

How does the label help the consumer?

- The label clearly identifies the active ingredient or ingredients.

- The label helps you compare products and choose the best one for your specific illness or condition.

- The labeling information helps you use the product correctly in order to get the maximum effect.

- Carefully reading the label will give you most of the information needed to avoid potential problems.

What is on the label?

ACTIVE INGREDIENTS

The active ingredient is the chemical compound in the medicine that works to relieve your symptoms. It is always the first item on the label. There may be more than one active ingredient in a product. The label will clearly show this, and it will also show the purpose of each active ingredient. It is usually best for breastfeeding individuals to take products with single active ingredients. Many different products can contain the same active ingredients. To reduce your risk and your baby's risk of overdose, check that you're not taking two medicines containing the same ingredients or intended for the same purpose.

Note: In the tables in this book, active ingredients will be listed for each product.

USES

This section lists the symptoms that the medicine is meant to treat. Uses are sometimes called "indications."

WARNINGS

This safety information will tell you which other medicines, foods, or activities (such as driving) to avoid while taking this medicine, as well as possible side effects of taking the medicine. The warnings will also tell you if the medicine is not recommended for a particular group of people, such as pregnant women.

DIRECTIONS

This section tells you how much medicine you should take, how often you should take it, and for how long you can take it. The directions may be different for children and adults.

OTHER INFORMATION

Any other important information, such as the appropriate way to store the medicine, will be listed here.

INACTIVE INGREDIENTS

An inactive ingredient is a chemical compound in the medicine that isn't meant to treat a symptom. This can include preservatives, binding agents, and food coloring. This section is especially important for people who know they and/or their babies have allergies to food coloring or other chemicals.

Note: Most inactive ingredients are NOT listed in this book. When taking a non-prescription drug, carefully read all ingredients on the label.

QUESTIONS OR COMMENTS

A toll-free number for the manufacturer is provided in case you have any questions or want to share your comments about the medicine.

The following label example is for an allergy relief product:

Drug Facts

Active ingredient	Purpose
Chlorpheniramine maleate 2 mg..Antihistamine	

Uses temporarily relieves these symptoms due to hay fever or other upper respiratory allergies:
■ sneezing   ■ runny nose   ■ itchy, watery eyes   ■ itchy throat

Warnings

Ask a doctor before use if you have ■ glaucoma
■ a breathing problem such as emphysema or chronic bronchitis
■ trouble urinating due to an enlarged prostate gland

When using this product
■ drowsiness may occur   ■ avoid alcoholic drinks
■ alcohol, sedatives, and tranquilizers may increase drowsiness
■ be careful when driving a motor vehicle or operating machinery
■ excitability may occur, especially in children

If pregnant or breastfeeding, ask a health professional before use.
Keep out of reach of children. In case of overdose, get medical help or contact a Poison Control Center right away.

Directions

adults and children 12 years and over	take 2 tablets every 4 to 6 hours; not more than 12 tablets in 24 hours
children 6 years to under 12 years	take 1 tablet every 4 to 6 hours; not more than 6 tablets in 24 hours

▼

Drug facts (continued)   ▲

Other Information   ■ store at 20-25° C (68-77° F)   ■ protect from moisture

Inactive ingredients D&C yellow no. 10, lactose, magnesium stearate, microcrystalline cellulose, pregelatinized starch

Questions or comments? 1-800-xxx-xxxx

How to Read the Tables in This Book

This book contains a series of tables that list commonly used nonprescription medications and their active ingredients; hygiene and skincare products; galactagogues and other herbals; dietary products; and social drugs including alcohol, caffeine, tobacco, marijuana, and CBD.

From these lists, you will be able to select a suitable product to treat your symptoms that will allow you to continue to breastfeed safely.

The tables and lists throughout this book provide qualified yes-or-no answers to whether or not a specific nonprescription preparation or active ingredient is safe for a breastfeeding parent to use.

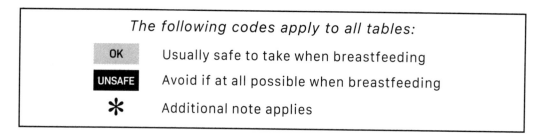

The following codes apply to all tables:

OK	Usually safe to take when breastfeeding
UNSAFE	Avoid if at all possible when breastfeeding
*	Additional note applies

If there are any additional notes about how to use a specific product safely, the note will be included in the table. All tables, products, and ingredients are organized in alphabetical order for easy reference.

Any nonprescription medications presented in the tables are designated as nonprescription or OTC in the United States. In other countries, some of these products may remain prescription drugs. Similarly, some drugs that must be prescribed in the U.S. can be purchased without a prescription in other countries. This book only addresses medications available without a prescription in the United States. Product names, dosage strengths, and forms may vary from country to country. The tables are not meant to be all-inclusive or comprehensive for all countries.

The tables also do not include information about whether the product or active ingredient is safe for use while breastfeeding premature or newborn (younger than one month) infants. In the very rare case where a product that is safe for older children is not safe for premature or newborn infants, a lactation consultant, healthcare provider, or knowledgeable pharmacist can let you know and help you find a suitable alternative.

Dr. Hale's Lactation Risk Categories

You will notice that each table entry throughout the book also has a safety rating of L1–L5. These ratings are referencing the Lactation Risk Categories created by Thomas W. Hale, R.Ph., Ph.D. They are also available at HaleMeds.com and have been used with permission.

L1 SAFEST:

The drug has been taken by a large number of breastfeeding mothers without any negative effects observed in the infants. Controlled studies show no risk or insignificant risk of harm.

L2 SAFER:

The drug has been taken by a limited number of breastfeeding mothers without any negative effects observed in the infants, and/or controlled studies show insignificant risk of harm.

L3 MODERATELY SAFE:

There are no controlled studies available, or controlled studies show minimal, non-threatening adverse effects. The drug should be used only if the potential benefit for the breastfeeding parent justifies the potential risk to the infant. **New medications that have no published data are automatically listed in this category, regardless of how safe or how dangerous they may be.**

L4 POSSIBLY HAZARDOUS:

Studies show increased risk of harm to breastfed infants, or a negative effect on breastmilk production. The benefit of the drug for the parent may justify the risk to the infant if the drug is needed in a life-threatening situation or to treat a serious disease for which safer drugs cannot be used or are ineffective.

L5 CONTRAINDICATED:

Studies among breastfeeding mothers have documented significant risk of harm to breastfed infants. The risk of using the drug clearly outweighs any benefit gained from breastfeeding. The drug is absolutely never recommended for anyone currently breastfeeding an infant.

What to Do When You Believe You or Your Baby May Be Experiencing a Side Effect

When you use any over-the-counter medication, herbal, or supplement, always read the WARNINGS section on the label and/or instructions that come with the product to see what possible common side effects may occur. Even when the product you are using is generally safe to use while breastfeeding, side effects are still possible. Fortunately, most are self-limiting and not serious.

You should always monitor both yourself and your breastfed baby for any potential side effects. These can include rashes (skin and diaper rash), irritability, diarrhea or constipation, gas, and others. Your pharmacist can advise you on which side effects are serious, which ones will go away on their own, and which ones can be prevented. Once you start taking a medication, mention any unexpected symptoms to your lactation consultant, pharmacist, and/or healthcare provider as soon as possible. Stop taking or using the medication if you have any doubts about its safety for you or your baby until you receive further professional advice.

If you have any concern about your child's breathing or mental state, call 911 immediately.

Side effects to watch for may also include a reduction in the amount of breastmilk your infant receives. Talk to a lactation consultant about strategies for monitoring your milk supply and your baby's breastmilk intake.

3.

ACTIVE INGREDIENTS

There are hundreds of active ingredients in both prescription and nonprescription drugs. Recognizing and understanding the active ingredients listed on the label of your OTC medications can be a great way for you to take control of your health and ensure that you are using the correct products. Anyone taking a nonprescription medication, especially those who are breastfeeding, should always read the active ingredients before using an OTC product.

The tables in this section describe whether or not the listed active ingredients are safe for breastfeeding. The tables will not describe which ingredients can be safely combined or the proper directions or dosage.

Remember:

- Avoid using OTC products with multiple active ingredients.

- Consumers should ask their pharmacist before combining products with different active ingredients.

- Avoid taking two different products that have one or more overlapping active ingredients (e.g., don't take DayQuil Cold + Flu and Tylenol at the same time because they both contain the active ingredient acetaminophen).

- Always follow instructions for nonprescription medications.

Directory of Active Ingredient Tables

For Localized Pain, Itching, or Inflammation:
Analgesics, Anesthetics, and Anti-Inflammatories (Topical)

Information Capsules:

 ANALGESICS (pain relievers) are probably the most common class of OTCs used by breastfeeding mothers.

 Products used for sore throats may contain a variety of soothing agents (**CAMPHOR, MENTHOL**) and local anesthetics (**DYCLONINE, BENZOCAINE**). The majority of these products are safe for use, since they are found minimally in breastmilk.

 PHENOL should be avoided, since safer alternatives are available.

		SAFETY LEVEL (PAGE 19)	DO NOT APPLY TO BREASTS
Aloe / Aloe vera	OK	L3	*
Apple cider vinegar	OK	L1	*
Arnica montana	OK	L3	*
Benzethonium chloride	OK	L1	*
Benzocaine	OK	L2	*
Bifidobacterium infantis	OK	L1	*
Bifidobacterium lactis	OK	L1	*
Budesonide	OK	L1	*
Cajuput oil	OK	L2	*
Calamine	OK	L3	*
Calendula / Pot marigold	OK	L1	*
Camphor	OK	L2	*
Camphorated phenol	UNSAFE	L4	
Candida albicans	OK	L3	*
Capsaicin	OK	L2	*

		SAFETY LEVEL (PAGE 19)	DO NOT APPLY TO BREASTS
Capsicum oleoresin	OK	L2	✳
Chamomile	OK	L2	✳
Chloroxylenol	OK	L2	✳
Clove oil	OK	L2	✳
Coriander seed	OK	L1	✳
Dibucaine	OK	L3	✳
Diclofenac sodium	OK	L2	✳
Diphenhydramine	OK	L2	✳
Dyclonine	OK	L3	✳
Elderberry	OK	L1	✳
Emu oil	OK	L3	✳
Eucalyptol	OK	L2	✳
Eucalyptus	OK	L2	✳
Eucalyptus leaf oil	OK	L1	✳
Ferrum phosphoricum	OK	L1	✳
Fluticasone	OK	L3	✳
Ginger	OK	L1	✳
Glucosamine	OK	L1	✳
Honey	OK	L1	✳
Hydrocortisone	OK	L2	✳
Ibuprofen	OK	L1	✳
Kreosotum	OK	L3	✳
Lactobacillus acidophilus	OK	L1	✳
Lidocaine	OK	L2	✳
Magnesium sulfate	OK	L1	✳
Menthol	OK	L1	✳
Methylsalicylate	OK	L3	✳
Methylsufonylmethane	OK	L1	✳
Mometasone	OK	L3	✳

		SAFETY LEVEL (PAGE 19)	DO NOT APPLY TO BREASTS
Natrum muriaticum	OK	L3	*
Nonoxynol-9	OK	L3	*
Pelargonium sidoides	OK	L3	*
Peppermint oil	OK	L1	*
Phenazone	OK	L2	*
Phenol	UNSAFE	L4	
Polyethylene granules	OK	L3	*
Potassium nitrate	OK	L1	*
Pramoxine	OK	L1	*
Silicon dioxide	OK	L3	*
Sodium lauroyl sarcosinate	OK	L3	*
Solanum dulcamara	OK	L3	*
Spearmint oil	OK	L2	*
Sulfur	OK	L3	*
Thymol	OK	L2	*
Triamcinolone	OK	L3	*
Trolamine salicylate	OK	L3	*
Turmeric	OK	L1	*
Vitamin C	OK	L1	*
Wintergreen oil	OK	L2	*
Zinc acetate	OK	L1	*

For General Pain, Swelling, and Fever:
Analgesics, Anti-Inflammatories, and Antipyretics (Oral)

Information Capsules:

 ASPIRIN can have a tendency to cause adverse effects in infants, especially if used at higher doses. Also, due to a possible link with Reye's syndrome, the use of aspirin and other salicylates in high doses is not recommended. However, aspirin at a low dose of 81 mg or 162 mg is often recommended for myocardial infarction (heart attack) and stroke risk prevention. Due to the chemical properties of aspirin at these low doses, the potential risk for Reye's syndrome developing in a breastfed infant should be nonexistent. As such, **LOW-DOSE ASPIRIN** is usually compatible with breastfeeding.

 IBUPROFEN is the Non-Steroidal Anti-Inflammatory Drug (NSAID) of choice and has the best breastfeeding safety profile among the NSAIDs. Possessing similar safety profiles, **KETOPROFEN** and **NAPROXEN** are considered usually safe NSAID alternatives during breastfeeding. Do not exceed recommended NSAID doses.

ACETAMINOPHEN (also called paracetamol) is an analgesic or pain reliever of choice for breastfeeding parents, since the amount of the drug that transfers to breastmilk is relatively small. Do not exceed recommended doses.

		SAFETY LEVEL (PAGE 19)
Acetaminophen	OK	L1
African geranium root	OK	L3
Agave	OK	L3
Allium cepa	OK	L3
Apis mellifica	OK	L3
Aspirin	UNSAFE	L4

		SAFETY LEVEL (PAGE 19)
Aspirin (low-dose)	OK	L3
Belladonna	UNSAFE	L4
Black carrot extract	OK	L3
Bryonia	OK	L3
Caffeine	OK	L1
Choline salicylate	UNSAFE	L4
Cranberry	OK	L1
Eupatorium perfoliatum	OK	L3
Gelsemium sempervirens	OK	L3
Ibuprofen	OK	L1
Ivy leaf	OK	L3
Ketoprofen	OK	L3
Magnesium salicylate	UNSAFE	L4
Naproxen	OK	L3
Paracetamol	OK	L1
Phenazopyridine	OK	L3
Salicylamide	UNSAFE	L4
Elderberry	OK	L1
Sodium salicylate	UNSAFE	L4
Zinc	OK	L2
Zinc gluconate	OK	L2
Zincum gluconicum	OK	L2

For Urinary Tract Infections:
Analgesics, Anti-Inflammatories, and Antipyretics (Oral)

		SAFETY LEVEL (PAGE 19)
Acetaminophen	OK	L1
Aspirin	UNSAFE	L4
Benzoic acid	OK	L1
Cranberry	OK	L1
D-mannose	OK	L1
Ibuprofen	OK	L1
Ketoprofen	OK	L3
Magnesium salicylate	UNSAFE	L4
Methenamine	OK	L3
Naproxen	OK	L3
Paracetamol	OK	L1
Phenazopyridine	OK	L3
Salicylamide	UNSAFE	L4
Sodium salicylate	UNSAFE	L4

For Heartburn or an Upset Stomach:
Antacids, Anti-Nausea, and Gastric Acid Reducers

Information Capsules:

 Antacids are considered safe because a breastfed infant is exposed to only small amounts of **CALCIUM**, **ALUMINUM**, **MAGNESIUM**, and/or **SODIUM** from breastmilk. They are unlikely to increase bodily concentrations of these minerals, and therefore toxic reactions are unlikely to occur.

 In general, all of the H2-antagonists (ingredients that reduce acid produced by cells in the stomach) like **CIMETIDINE**, **FAMOTIDINE**, **NIZATIDINE**, and **RANITIDINE** are considered safe for use. However, famotidine and nizatidine are the preferred H2-antagonists to be used by breastfeeding parents because these are found in lower concentrations in breastmilk than cimetidine and ranitidine.

 Any **OMEPRAZOLE** (for frequent heartburn) ingested through breast-milk should be neutralized in the infant's digestive system, and is therefore safe.

 COLA SYRUP and **PHOSPHORATED CARBOHYDRATE** preparations are excellent choices to treat nausea and vomiting while breastfeeding.

		SAFETY LEVEL (PAGE 19)
Aluminum carbonate	OK	L1
Aluminum hydroxide	OK	L1
Aluminum trihydroxide	OK	L1
Birch	OK	L3
Bismuth subsalicylate	UNSAFE	L4
Calcium	OK	L1
Calcium carbonate	OK	L1
Cellulose gum	OK	L3
Chamomile	OK	L1

		SAFETY LEVEL (PAGE 19)
Cimetidine	OK	L2
Cola syrup	OK	L1
Dimethicone	OK	L3
Esomeprazole	OK	L2
Famotidine	OK	L2
Frankincense	OK	L3
Ginger	OK	L1
Hypromellose	OK	L1
Lansoprazole	OK	L2
Lavender	OK	L3
Magaldrate	OK	L1
Magnesium carbonate	OK	L1
Magnesium hydroxide	OK	L1
Magnesium oxide	OK	L1
Magnesium stearate	OK	L1
Magnesium stearatitanium dioxide	OK	L1
Magnesium trihydroxide	OK	L1
Maltodextrin	OK	L1
Microcrystalline cellulose	OK	L3
Myrrh	OK	L3
Nizatidine	OK	L2
Omeprazole	OK	L2
Phosphorated carbohydrates	OK	L1
Potassium bicarbonate	OK	L1
Ranitidine	OK	L2
Silicon dioxide	OK	L3
Sodium bicarbonate	OK	L1
Sodium hyaluronate	OK	L1
Soy	OK	L1
Ylang ylang	UNSAFE	L4

For Diarrhea:

Antidiarrheals

Information Capsules:

 Small amounts of **LOPERAMIDE** may be found in breastmilk, but appear to have no effect on infants. The use of loperamide should not exceed two days for the treatment of diarrhea.

 ATTAPULGITE is safe for infants to ingest through breastmilk since it is not absorbed from the gastrointestinal tract.

 The use of **BISMUTH SUBSALICYLATE** is not recommended. It has been investigated in infants and young children with watery diarrhea, and while the amount found in breastmilk should be compatible with nursing, there is an unknown risk associated with salicylates and the development of Reye's syndrome.

		SAFETY LEVEL (PAGE 19)	DO NOT USE MORE THAN 2 DAYS
Attapulgite	OK	L1	
Bismuth subsalicylate	UNSAFE	L4	
Calcium polycarbophil	OK	L1	
Loperamide	OK	L2	*
Pectin	OK	L1	

For Gas:
Antiflatulents

Information Capsules:

 Antiflatulents (for treatment of excessive gas) containing **SIMETHICONE** and **LACTASE** are considered safe for use.

 SIMETHICONE is not absorbed readily by the gastrointestinal tract, meaning only very small amounts of the drug would appear in breastmilk. Simethicone is also regularly used in colicky infants.

 LACTASE is a supplemental enzyme used for lactose intolerance.

		SAFETY LEVEL (PAGE 19)
Activated charcoal	OK	L1
Lactase	OK	L1
Lactobacillus acidophilus	OK	L1
Simethicone	OK	L1

For Yeast Infection or Thrush:
Antifungals and Probiotics

Information Capsules:

 Vaginal products used for candidiasis usually contain ingredients such as **NYSTATIN, MICONAZOLE, FLUCONAZOLE** and **CLOTRIMAZOLE**, which have not been shown to cause adverse effects when passed to an infant through breastmilk. OTC products containing these ingredients can also be used topically to treat nipple thrush.

 GRAPEFRUIT SEED EXTRACT (GSE) is a good natural alternative or additional supplement to treat nipple thrush. It can be used topically or taken in capsule form. Do not confuse with grape seed extract.

		SAFETY LEVEL (PAGE 19)	DO NOT APPLY TO BREASTS	IF APPLIED TO NIPPLE, WIPE OFF BEFORE FEEDING
Bifidobacterium infantis	OK	L1	*	
Bifidobacterium lactis	OK	L1	*	
Clotrimazole	OK	L1		*
D-mannose	OK	L1		*
Fluconazole	OK	L2		*
Grapefruit seed extract	OK	L1		*
Jojoba oil	OK	L3		*
Kreosotum	OK	L3		*
Lactic acid	OK	L1		*
Lactobacillus acidophilus	OK	L1	*	
Lactoferrin	OK	L1		*
Miconazole	OK	L2		*
Natrum muriaticum	OK	L3	*	
Nystatin	OK	L2		*
Tioconazole	OK	L2		*

For Allergies or Insect Bites:
Antihistamines

Information Capsules:

 Overall, antihistamines (allergy blockers) are reasonably safe to use while breastfeeding.

 It is best to take antihistamines at bedtime after breastfeeding because they may cause irritability or drowsiness in infants. Also, avoid long-acting, combination, or high-dose antihistamines to help lessen these side effects.

 The use of antihistamines for nausea and motion sickness, such as **DIPHENHYDRAMINE** and **DIMENHYDRINATE**, is usually safe to use while breastfeeding. Infants should be monitored for irritability and/or drowsiness with the use of these antihistamines.

 Avoid **MECLIZINE** and **CYCLIZINE** as long as other alternatives are available. There is limited information on the use of cyclizine and meclizine in nursing mothers.

		SAFETY LEVEL (PAGE 19)	MONITOR INFANT FOR DROWSINESS
Cetirizine	OK	L2	*
Chlorpheniramine	OK	L3	*
Clemastine	UNSAFE	L4	
Cromolyn sodium	OK	L3	*
Cyclizine	OK	L3	*
Dimenhydrinate	OK	L2	*
Diphenhydramine	OK	L2	*
Doxylamine	OK	L3	*
Fexofenadine	OK	L2	*
Ketotifen	OK	L3	*
Loratadine	OK	L2	*

* *Additional note applies*   35   OK *OK to use*   UNSAFE *Do not use*

		SAFETY LEVEL (PAGE 19)	MONITOR INFANT FOR DROWSINESS
Meclizine	OK	L3	*
Olopatidine	OK	L2	*
Pheniramine	OK	L3	*
Phenyltoloxamine	OK	L3	*
Pramoxine	OK	L3	*
Pyrilamine	OK	L3	*
Triprolidine	OK	L1	*

For Bacterial, Fungal, and Parasitic Infections, for Skin/Face Cleansers and Oral Hygiene, or for Disinfecting Cuts, Burns, and Bites:

Anti-Infectives, Antifungals, Antiseptics, and Astringents (Topical)

Information Capsules:

🔖 Products used for sore throats may contain a variety of antiseptics like **ALLANTOIN**. The majority of these products are safe for use, since they are found minimally in breastmilk.

		SAFETY LEVEL (PAGE 19)	DO NOT APPLY TO BREASTS	IF APPLIED TO NIPPLE, WIPE OFF BEFORE FEEDING	AVOID BREATHING IN FUMES
8-hydroxyquinolone	OK	L2	*		
Acetic acid	OK	L1	*		
Acrylate terpolymer	OK	L3	*		*
Adapalene	OK	L3	*		
Aesculus hippocastanum	OK	L3	*		
Allantoin	OK	L1	*		
Allium sativum	OK	L1	*		
Aluminum sulfate	OK	L1	*		
Bacitracin	OK	L2		*	
Bacitracin zinc	OK	L2		*	
Baking soda	OK	L1	*		
Barberry	OK	L1		*	
Benzalkonium chloride	OK	L1	*		
Benzethonium chloride	OK	L1	*		
Benzocaine	OK	L2	*		
Benzoic acid	OK	L1	*		

		SAFETY LEVEL (PAGE 19)	DO NOT APPLY TO BREASTS	IF APPLIED TO NIPPLE, WIPE OFF BEFORE FEEDING	AVOID BREATHING IN FUMES
Benzoyl peroxide	OK	L1	*		
Benzyl alcohol	OK	L1	*		
Boric acid	OK	L1	*		
Butenafine	OK	L2	*		
Calcarea fluorica	OK	L3	*		
Calcium acetate	OK	L1	*		
Camphor	OK	L1	*		
Carbamide peroxide	OK	L1	*		
Cedar oil	OK	L3	*		
Ceresin	OK	L1	*		
Cetyl alcohol	OK	L2	*		
Cetylpyridium	OK	L1	*		
Chlorhexidine	UNSAFE	L4			
Chloroxylenol	OK	L2	*		
Citric acid	OK	L1	*		
Citronella oil	OK	L3	*		
Citroxain	OK	L2	*		
Clotrimazole	OK	L1		*	
Coal tar	OK	L3	*		*
Cocamidopropyl betaine	OK	L3		*	
Coco betaine	OK	L3		*	
Dimethyl ether-propane	OK	L2	*		*
Docosanol	OK	L2	*		
Emu oil	OK	L2	*		
Ethyl alcohol	OK	L3	*		*
Eugenol	OK	L2	*		
Fluconazole	OK	L2		*	
Fluoride	OK	L1	*		

		SAFETY LEVEL (PAGE 19)	DO NOT APPLY TO BREASTS	IF APPLIED TO NIPPLE, WIPE OFF BEFORE FEEDING	AVOID BREATHING IN FUMES
Gamma-hexachlorocyclohexane	UNSAFE	L4			
Geraniol	OK	L3	*		
Hexamethyldisiloxane	OK	L3	*		*
Hexetidine	OK	L2	*		
Hydantoin	OK	L1	*		
Hydrogen peroxide	OK	L1	*		
Ichthammol	OK	L1	*		*
Isopropyl alcohol	OK	L2	*		*
Ketoconazole	OK	L2		*	
Kreosotum	OK	L1		*	
Lemongrass oil	OK	L2		*	
Lindane	UNSAFE	L4			
Lysine	OK	L1	*		
Magnesium peroxide	OK	L1	*		
Mercurius solubilus	OK	L3	*		
Methane oxybis	OK	L3	*		*
Miconazole	OK	L2		*	
Mountain grape root	OK	L1		*	
Natrum muriaticum	OK	L3	*		
Natural oil extracts	OK	L1	*		
Neomycin	OK	L2		*	
Nux vomica	OK	L3	*		
Nystatin	OK	L2		*	
Peppermint oil	OK	L1	*		
Permethrin	OK	L2	*		
Phytolacca decandra	OK	L3	*		
Piperonyl butoxide	OK	L2	*		
Polymyxin B	OK	L2		*	

* *Additional note applies*   39   OK *OK to use*   UNSAFE *Do not use*

		SAFETY LEVEL (PAGE 19)	DO NOT APPLY TO BREASTS	IF APPLIED TO NIPPLE, WIPE OFF BEFORE FEEDING	AVOID BREATHING IN FUMES
Polyphenylmethylsiloxane polymer	OK	L3	*		*
Potassium nitrate	OK	L1	*		
Povidone iodine (topical)	OK	L1	*		
Povidone iodine (vaginal use)	UNSAFE	L4			
Pyrantel pamoate	OK	L3		*	
Pyrethrum extract	OK	L2	*		
Pyrithione zinc	OK	L2	*		
Quaternary ammonium compounds	OK	L3	*		
Ratanhia peruviana	OK	L3	*		
Rosemary oil	OK	L2	*		
Salicylic acid	OK	L2	*		
Selenium sulfide	OK	L2	*		
Sesame oil	OK	L1	*		
Silicon dioxide	OK	L1	*		
Sodium borate	OK	L1	*		
Sodium fluoride	OK	L1	*		
Sodium oxychlorosene	OK	L3	*		
Sodium perborate monohydrate	OK	L1	*		
Stannous fluoride	OK	L1	*		
Stearyl alcohol	OK	L2	*		
Stevia rebaudiana	OK	L3	*		
Stone root	OK	L1		*	
Sulfur	OK	L2	*		
Terbinafine	OK	L2		*	
Tetrasodium pyrophosphate	OK	L1	*		
Thuja occidentalis	OK	L3	*		
Tioconazole	OK	L2		*	
Tolnaftate	OK	L2		*	

3. ACTIVE INGREDIENTS   Anti-Infectives, Antifungals, Antiseptics, and Astringents (Topical)

		SAFETY LEVEL (PAGE 19)	DO NOT APPLY TO BREASTS	IF APPLIED TO NIPPLE, WIPE OFF BEFORE FEEDING	AVOID BREATHING IN FUMES
Triclosan	OK	L1	✳		
Undecylenic acid	OK	L1	✳		
Vinegar	OK	L1	✳		
Zinc	OK	L1	✳		
Zinc acetate	OK	L1	✳		
Zinc chloride	OK	L1	✳		
Zinc sulfate	OK	L1	✳		
Zincum oxydatum	UNSAFE	L4			

 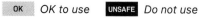

For a Cough:
Antitussives and Expectorants

Information Capsules:

 GUAIFENESIN (expectorant to loosen phlegm) and **DEXTROMETHO-RPHAN** (antitussive to suppress cough) at recommended doses have had no reported adverse effects in breastfed infants.

		SAFETY LEVEL (PAGE 19)	MONITOR INFANT FOR DROWSINESS OR EXCITABILITY
Dextromethorphan	OK	L1	✳
Guaifenesin	OK	L2	
Menthol	OK	L1	
Potassium guaiacolsulfonate	OK	L2	
Potassium iodide	UNSAFE	L4	

For a Stuffy Nose or Sinus Pressure:
Decongestants

Information Capsules:

 Decongestants, especially if they are used after six months postpartum, may cause a decrease in breastmilk production. Drinking extra fluids can help remedy this.

 Decongestants in most cold medications include **PSEUDOEPHEDRINE** or **PHENYLEPHRINE**. After taking these drugs, only small amounts of pseudoephedrine can be found in breastmilk, and insignificant amounts of phenylephrine have been reported.

 Products containing **PSEUDOEPHEDRINE** are only sold from behind a pharmacy or service counter, even when they do not require a prescription. Products with **PHENYLEPHRINE** are less effective, but more easily available.

 While **NAPHAZOLINE**, **OXYMETAZOLINE**, and **XYLOMETAZOLINE** are very effective, they are also long-acting. These products should not be used for more than three to four days in a row, and it is important to monitor milk supply.

 PHENYLEPHRINE is not as long-acting as other nasal decongestants. It is usually safe for breastfeeding; however, it is still important to monitor milk supply.

	SAFETY LEVEL (PAGE 19)		MONITOR INFANT FOR DROWSINESS OR EXCITABILITY	MONITOR MILK SUPPLY & DRINK EXTRA FLUIDS
Antazoline	OK	L3	✳	✳
Levmetamfetamine	OK	L3	✳	✳
Naphazoline	OK	L3	✳	✳
Oxymetazoline	OK	L3	✳	✳

		SAFETY LEVEL (PAGE 19)	MONITOR INFANT FOR DROWSINESS OR EXCITABILITY	MONITOR MILK SUPPLY & DRINK EXTRA FLUIDS
Phenylephrine	OK	L3	*	*
Propylhexedrine	UNSAFE	L5		
Pseudoephedrine	OK	L3	*	*
Tetrahydrozoline	OK	L3	*	*
Xylometazoline	OK	L3	*	*

For Lowering Blood Pressure and Reducing Swelling or Bloating:
Diuretics

Information Capsules:

 PAMABROM is a bromide-containing product with no adequate, well-controlled studies or case reports on its safety for breastfeeding individuals. It is not recommended.

		SAFETY LEVEL (PAGE 19)
Pamabrom	UNSAFE	L4

For Constipation:
Laxatives and Stool Softeners

Information Capsules:

 Laxatives are generally considered safe in breastfeeding, and bulk-forming laxatives (**PSYLLIUM**, **METHYLCELLULOSE**, etc.) can be considered first line agents for constipation. These agents are not absorbed from the gastrointestinal tract, and as a result, do not enter the infant's circulation.

 Limit use of **SENNA**-containing products to one or two days at a time.

 No adverse effects have been reported with **DOCUSATE**, a stool softening agent.

GLYCERIN suppositories, **MAGNESIUM CITRATE**, and **SODIUM BIPHOSPHATE-PHOSPHATE** enemas are also safe for use.

		SAFETY LEVEL (PAGE 19)	DO NOT USE FOR MORE THAN 1–2 DOSES
Bisacodyl	OK	L2	*
Calcium polycarbophil	OK	L2	
Cascara sagrada	UNSAFE	L3	
Castor oil	UNSAFE	L3	
Chicory root fiber	OK	L1	
Dibasic sodium phosphate	OK	L1	*
Docusate calcium	OK	L2	
Docusate sodium	OK	L2	
Glycerin	OK	L1	*
Hydroxycellulose	OK	L1	
Magnesium citrate	OK	L1	*
Magnesium hydroxide	OK	L1	
Methylcellulose	OK	L1	

		SAFETY LEVEL (PAGE 19)	DO NOT USE FOR MORE THAN 1–2 DOSES
Mineral oil	OK	L1	✳
Monobasic sodium phosphate	OK	L1	✳
PEG-3350	OK	L3	✳
Picosulphate	OK	L3	✳
Potassium bitartrate	OK	L1	✳
Potassium sorbate	OK	L1	✳
Psyllium	OK	L1	
Rhubarb root	UNSAFE	L4	
Saline	OK	L1	✳
Senna	OK	L3	✳
Sennosides	OK	L3	✳
Sodium propionate	OK	L1	✳
Sorbitol	OK	L1	
Wheat dextrin	OK	L1	

For Dryness, Chafing, Itching, and Burns:
Lubricants, Moisturizers, and Protectants

		SAFETY LEVEL (PAGE 19)	WASH OFF NIPPLE AREA WITH SOAP & WATER BEFORE BREASTFEEDING
Acacia gum	OK	L1	*
Aloe / Aloe vera	OK	L1	*
Aminobenzoic acid	OK	L1	*
Ammonium lactate	OK	L1	*
Angelica root	OK	L3	*
Avobenzone	OK	L1	*
Avocado oil	OK	L3	*
Beeswax	OK	L1	*
Bentoquatam	OK	L2	*
Benzophenone-9	OK	L1	*
Betaine / trimethylglycine	OK	L2	*
Bisabolol	OK	L3	*
Calcium carbonate	OK	L1	*
Calendula	OK	L2	*
Canola oil	OK	L1	*
Caprylic / capric triglyceride	OK	L1	*
Carbamide peroxide	OK	L1	*
Carboxymethylcellulose	OK	L1	*
Carnosine	OK	L1	*
Castor oil	OK	L1	*
Cellulose gum	OK	L1	*
Centella asiatica	OK	L1	*
Ceramides	OK	L1	*
Cetearyl alcohol	OK	L1	*
Chamomile	OK	L1	*

		SAFETY LEVEL (PAGE 19)	WASH OFF NIPPLE AREA WITH SOAP & WATER BEFORE BREASTFEEDING
Cinoxate	OK	L1	*
Cocamidopropyl betaine	OK	L3	*
Coco betaine	OK	L3	*
Cocoa butter / kokum butter	OK	L1	*
Cod liver oil	OK	L1	*
Colloidal oatmeal	OK	L1	*
Compound benzoin tincture	OK	L1	*
Corn starch	OK	L1	*
Dextran	OK	L1	*
Dimethicone	OK	L2	*
Dioxybenzone	OK	L1	*
Ecamsule	OK	L1	*
Echinacea	OK	L1	*
Giant kelp leaf extract	OK	L1	*
Ginger	OK	L1	*
Glycerin / glycerine / glycerol	OK	L1	*
Glycogen	OK	L1	*
Grapefruit seed extract	OK	L1	*
Guava	OK	L1	*
Hamamelis	OK	L1	*
Homosalate	OK	L1	*
Hyaluronic acid	OK	L1	*
Hydroxyethylcellulose	OK	L1	*
Hydroxypropyl methylcellulose	OK	L1	*
Hypromellose	OK	L1	*
Imidazolidinyl urea	OK	L1	*
Isopentyl-4-methoxycinnamate	OK	L1	*
Jojoba	OK	L3	*
Jojoba oil	OK	L3	*

		SAFETY LEVEL (PAGE 19)	WASH OFF NIPPLE AREA WITH SOAP & WATER BEFORE BREASTFEEDING
Lactic acid	OK	L1	✳
Lactoferrin	OK	L1	✳
Lanolin	OK	L1	✳
Lanolin oil	OK	L1	✳
Magnesium stearate	OK	L1	✳
Mango butter	OK	L1	✳
Mannose	OK	L1	✳
Methyl anthranilate	OK	L1	✳
Methylbenzylidene camphor	OK	L1	✳
Mexoryl XL	OK	L1	✳
Mineral oil	OK	L1	✳
Myrcia oil	OK	L1	✳
Neo Heliopan AP	OK	L1	✳
Oat kernel extract	OK	L1	✳
Oat kernel flour / colloidal oat flour	OK	L1	✳
Octocrylene	OK	L1	✳
Octyl methoxycinnamate	OK	L1	✳
Octyl salicylate	OK	L1	✳
Olive oil	OK	L1	✳
Onion extract	OK	L1	✳
Oxybenzone	OK	L1	✳
PABA	OK	L1	✳
Padimate O	OK	L1	✳
Papaya	OK	L1	✳
Paraffin	OK	L1	✳
Parsol SLX	OK	L1	✳
Passion fruit oil	OK	L1	✳
PEG-6-32	OK	L1	✳
PEG-20	OK	L1	✳

		SAFETY LEVEL (PAGE 19)	WASH OFF NIPPLE AREA WITH SOAP & WATER BEFORE BREASTFEEDING
PEG-40	OK	L1	*
PEG-400	OK	L1	*
PEG-8000	OK	L1	*
Peruvian balsam	OK	L1	*
Petrolatum	OK	L1	*
Phenylbenzimidazole sulfonic acid	OK	L1	*
Plumeria	OK	L1	*
Poloxamer 407	OK	L1	*
Polycarbophil	OK	L1	*
Polysorbate 80	OK	L1	*
Polyvinyl alcohol	OK	L1	*
Polyvinylpyrrolidone	OK	L1	*
Potassium lactate	OK	L1	*
Propylene glycol	OK	L1	*
Rebiana	OK	L3	*
Shark liver oil	OK	L1	*
Shea butter	OK	L1	*
Silicone	OK	L1	*
Sodium bicarbonate	OK	L1	*
Sodium chloride	OK	L1	*
Sodium hyaluronate	OK	L1	*
Sodium lactate	OK	L1	*
Sodium monofluorophosphate	OK	L2	*
Sorbitol	OK	L1	*
Starch	OK	L1	*
Sulisobenzone	OK	L1	*
Sunflower oil	OK	L1	*
Sweet almond oil	OK	L3	*
Taurine	OK	L1	*

		SAFETY LEVEL (PAGE 19)	WASH OFF NIPPLE AREA WITH SOAP & WATER BEFORE BREASTFEEDING
Tinosorb M	OK	L1	✳
Tinosorb S	OK	L1	✳
Titanium oxide	OK	L1	✳
Topical starch	OK	L1	✳
Trolamine salicylate	OK	L1	✳
Urea	OK	L1	✳
Uvasorb HEB	OK	L1	✳
Uvinul A Plus	OK	L1	✳
Uvinul T 150	OK	L1	✳
Vitamin A	OK	L1	✳
Vitamin D	OK	L1	✳
Vitamin E	OK	L1	✳
White petrolatum	OK	L1	✳
Witch hazel	OK	L1	✳
Xylitol	OK	L1	✳
Zinc gluconate	OK	L1	✳
Zinc oxide	OK	L1	✳

For Difficulty Sleeping:
Sleep Aids

Information Capsules:

 Most of the currently available sleep aid products contain **DIPHEN-HYDRAMINE**. The use of diphenhydramine has been shown to be usually safe and compatible with breastfeeding. Infants should still be monitored for irritability and/or drowsiness.

 Parents with autoimmune disorders, diabetes, and/or depression should avoid using **MELATONIN**.

		SAFETY LEVEL (PAGE 19)	MONITOR INFANT FOR DROWSINESS OR EXCITABILITY	TOTAL DOSE OF 1 mg TO 3 mg PER DAY
Bromelain	OK	L1		
Chamomile	OK	L1		
Diphenhydramine	OK	L2	*	
Doxylamine	OK	L3	*	
Lemon	OK	L1		
Lemon Balm	OK	L1		
Melatonin	OK	L3		*

For Quitting Tobacco Use:
Smoking Cessation Aids

		SAFETY LEVEL (PAGE 19)	FOLLOW DIRECTIONS EXPLICITLY	DO NOT SMOKE IN ADDITION TO USING THE INGREDIENT
Nicotine	OK	L1	*	*
Nicotine polacrilex	OK	L1	*	*

For Sun Protection:
Sunscreen Agents

Information Capsules:

 For **ALL PRODUCTS CONTAINING SUNSCREEN**, read the labels and do not use sunscreen agents exceeding their maximum percent concentrations listed below.

 Please note, sunscreens with a high Sun Protection Factor (SPF) will have a higher percent concentration, but the numbers are not equivalent. A 15% concentration does not equal 15 SPF. The SPF of the product depends on the ingredient(s) used as well as the percent concentration of each ingredient. Look for the active ingredients on the label in order to find the percent concentration.

 If applied to the nipple or areola, clean the area with warm water and mild soap before breastfeeding.

	MAXIMUM % CONCENTRATION		SAFETY LEVEL (PAGE 19)
Aminobenzoic acid (PABA)	15%	OK	L1
Avobenzone	3%	OK	L1
Benzophenone-9	10%	OK	L1
Cinoxate	3%	OK	L1
Dioxybenzone	3%	OK	L1
Ecamsule	3%	OK	L1
Homosalate	15%	OK	L1
Isopentenyl-4-methoxycinnamate	10%	OK	L1
Methyl anthranilate	5%	OK	L1
Methylbenzylidene camphor	4%	OK	L1
Mexoryl XL	15%	OK	L1
Neo Heliopan AP	10%	OK	L1

	MAXIMUM % CONCENTRATION		SAFETY LEVEL (PAGE 19)
Octocrylene	10%	OK	L1
Octyl methoxycinnamate	7.5%	OK	L1
Octyl salicylate	5%	OK	L1
Oxybenzone	6%	OK	L1
Padimate O	8%	OK	L1
Parsol SLX	10%	OK	L1
Phenylbenzimidazole sulfonic acid	4%	OK	L1
Sulisobenzone	10%	OK	L1
Tinosorb M	10%	OK	L1
Tinosorb S	10%	OK	L1
Titanium dioxide	25%	OK	L1
Trolamine salicylate	12%	OK	L1
Uvasorb HEB	10%	OK	L1
Uvinul A Plus	10%	OK	L1
Uvinul T 150	5%	OK	L1
Zinc oxide	25%	OK	L1

4.

FINDING THE RIGHT PRODUCT

Most Commonly Recommended Over-the-Counter Products

To make it easier and quicker to pick out safe products and locate information, the following section contains breastfeeding-compatible lists of the most commonly recommended over-the-counter products for each major drug category. The categories are derived from an annual survey conducted by *Pharmacy Times*, but the lists have been updated to exclude products that are no longer available or are unsafe for breastfeeding.

Each product category is organized by the symptom it is meant to treat and the form of the preparation. It will list the top brands or product lines that might be recommended to treat that symptom.

Question:

Which generic ingredient (not a brand) is most commonly used by consumers?

Answer:

Acetaminophen. It is found in over 600 different medications, the most popular being Tylenol. The total global acetaminophen market is estimated to be worth over $9 billion.

Directory of Product Lists: Most Commonly Recommended Breastfeeding-Safe Products

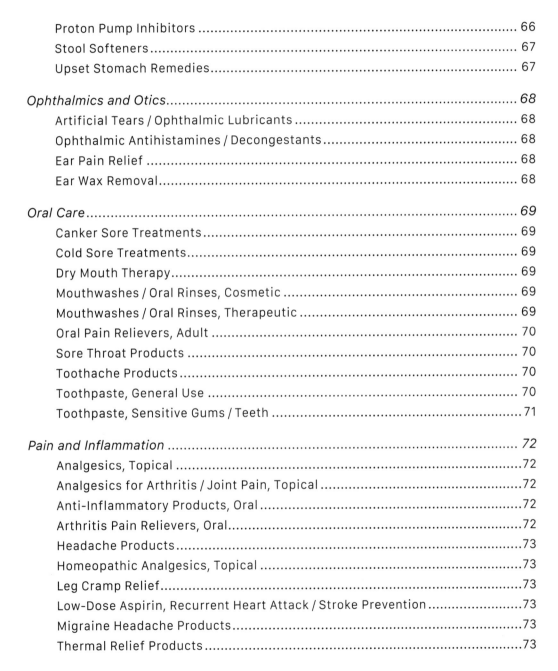

continued ›

Directory of Product Lists (continued)

Most Commonly Recommended Breastfeeding-Safe Products

The products or brands in each category are numbered in order of how often they are recommended by pharmacists.

Allergy, Cold, and Cough

Antihistamines, Oral
1. Claritin (see page 92 for more information)
2. Zyrtec (see page 100 for more information)
3. Allegra Allergy (see page 91 for more information)
4. Benadryl (see page 91 for more information)

Cold Remedies
1. Cepacol (see page 112 for more information)
2. Zicam RapidMelts (see page 100 for more information)
3. Cold-EEZE (see pages 92 and 112 for more information)
4. HALLS Defense (see page 112 for more information)
5. Airborne (see page 89 for more information)
6. Sucrets (see page 113 for more information)
7. Umcka ColdCare (see page 98 for more information)

Cold / Cough / Flu Combinations, Daytime
1. Vicks DayQuil (see page 99 for more information)
2. Advil Cold & Sinus (see page 89 for more information)
3. Mucinex (see page 94 for more information)
4. Tylenol Cold Max (see page 97 for more information)
5. TheraFlu (see page 97 for more information)
6. Claritin (see page 92 for more information)
7. Coricidin HBP (see page 93 for more information)
8. Sambucol (see pages 95 and 113 for more information)
9. Sudafed PE (phenylephrine) (see page 96 for more information)

Cold / Cough / Flu Combinations, Nighttime
1. Vicks NyQuil (see pages 99 and 100 for more information)

2. Delsym Nighttime (see page 93 for more information)
3. TheraFlu Nighttime (see page 97 for more information)
4. Coricidin HBP Nighttime (see page 93 for more information)
5. Robitussin Nighttime (see page 95 for more information)
6. Tylenol Nighttime (see page 98 for more information)
7. Contac Cold & Flu Night (see page 92 for more information)

Cough Suppressants

1. Delsym (see page 93 for more information)
2. Mucinex DM (see page 94 for more information)
3. Robitussin (see pages 94 and 95 for more information)
4. Vicks NyQuil (see pages 99 and 100 for more information)

Cough Suppressants, Safe For Diabetes

1. Diabetic Tussin (see pages 93 and 94 for more information)
2. Robitussin (see page 94 for more information)
3. Safetussin (see page 95 for more information)

Decongestants, Nasal Spray

1. Afrin (see page 125 for more information)
2. NasalCrom (see page 126 for more information)
3. NeilMed SinuFrin Plus (see page 126 for more information)
4. Neo-Synephrine (see page 126 for more information)
5. Vicks Sinex Ultra Fine Mist (see page 127 for more information)
6. Dristan Nasal Spray (see page 125 for more information)

Decongestants, Oral

1. Sudafed (pseudoephedrine) (see page 97 for more information)
2. Claritin-D (see page 92 for more information)
3. Allegra-D (see page 91 for more information)
4. Sudafed PE (phenylephrine) (see page 96 for more information)
5. Mucinex D (see page 94 for more information)
6. Zyrtec D (see page 100 for more information)
7. Advil Cold & Sinus (see page 89 for more information)

Decongestants, Oral (Abuse-Deterrent)

1. Zephrex-D (see page 100 for more information)
2. Nexafed (see page 94 for more information)

Expectorants

1. Mucinex (see page 94 for more information)
2. Robitussin (see pages 94 and 95 for more information)

Flu Products

1. TheraFlu (see page 97 for more information)
2. Vicks DayQuil Cold & Flu (see page 99 for more information)
3. Coricidin HBP Cold & Flu (see page 93 for more information)
4. Tylenol Cold & Flu Severe (see page 98 for more information)
5. Vicks Nyquil Cold & Flu (see pages 99 and 100 for more information)

Homeopathic Cold Products

1. Sambucol (see pages 95 and 113 for more information)

Homeopathic Cough Products

1. Sambucol Lozenges (see page 113 for more information)
2. Boiron Chestal (see page 92 for more information)
3. Umcka ColdCare (see page 98 for more information)

Homeopathic Flu Products

1. Sambucol Cold & Flu Relief (see page 95 for more information)
2. Umcka Cold + Flu (see page 98 for more information)

Intranasal Corticosteroids

1. Flonase Allergy Relief (see page 125 for more information)
2. Nasacort Allergy 24 HR (see page 126 for more information)

Saline Nasal Moisturizers

1. Arm & Hammer Simply Saline (see page 125 for more information)
2. Ayr (see page 125 for more information)
3. NeilMed NasalMist (see page 126 for more information)
4. SinuCleanse Nasal Wash (see page 127 for more information)
5. Xlear (see page 127 for more information)

Topical Cough Suppressant / Lozenges

1. Cepacol (see page 112 for more information)
2. HALLS (see page 112 for more information)
3. Chloraseptic (lozenges only) (see page 112 for more information)

4. Fisherman's Friend (see page 112 for more information)
5. Zarbee's Honey Cough Soothers (see page 113 for more information)
6. Luden's (see page 112 for more information)
7. Burt's Bees (see page 112 for more information)
8. Pine Brothers (see page 112 for more information)
9. Sucrets (see page 113 for more information)

Topical Vapor Therapy
1. Vicks (see page 113 for more information)
2. Maty's All Natural (see page 112 for more information)

Zinc Lozenges
1. Zicam (see page 113 for more information)
2. Cold-EEZE (see page 112 for more information)
3. Nature's Way (see page 112 for more information)
4. TheraZinc (see page 113 for more information)

Zinc Cold Remedies
1. Zicam RapidMelts (see pages 100 for more information)
2. Cold-EEZE (see pages 92 and 112 for more information)

Gastrointestinal

Acid Reducers

1. Pepcid (see page 107 for more information)
2. Prilosec OTC (see page 108 for more information)
3. Nexium 24 HR (see page 107 for more information)
4. Prevacid 24 HR (see page 107 for more information)
5. Zantac (see page 108 for more information)
6. Zegerid OTC (see page 108 for more information)

Antacids

1. TUMS (see page 108 for more information)
2. Gaviscon (see page 106 for more information)
3. Mylanta (see page 107 for more information)
4. Rolaids (see page 108 for more information)
5. Gelusil (see page 107 for more information)

Antidiarrheals

1. Imodium (see page 109 for more information)

Antiflatulents

1. Gas-X (see page 106 for more information)
2. Phazyme (see page 107 for more information)
3. Beano (see page 106 for more information)
4. Mylanta (see page 107 for more information)
5. CharcoCaps (see page 106 for more information)
6. Gelusil (see page 107 for more information)

H2-Receptor Antagonists

1. Pepcid (see page 107 for more information)
2. Tagamet HB 200 (see page 108 for more information)
3. Zantac (see page 108 for more information)

Lactose Intolerance Products

1. Lactaid (see page 107 for more information)
2. Beano (see page 106 for more information)
3. Nature's Way Lactase Enzyme (see page 107 for more information)
4. Schiff's Digestive Advantage (see page 108 for more information)

Laxatives, Bulk / Fiber

1. Metamucil (see pages 119 and 122 for more information)
2. Benefiber (see page 121 for more information)
3. Citrucel (see pages 118 and 121 for more information)
4. FiberCon (see pages 109, 118, and 122 for more information)

Laxatives, Nonfiber

1. MiraLAX (see page 122 for more information)
2. Dulcolax (see page 121 for more information)
3. Fleet (see page 122 for more information)
4. Phillips' (see page 122 for more information)

Laxatives, Stimulant

1. Dulcolax (see page 121 for more information)
2. Senokot (see pages 122 and 123 for more information)
3. Colace 2-in-1 (Peri-Colace) (see page 121 for more information)
4. Fleet (see page 122 for more information)
5. Ex-Lax (see page 122 for more information)

Motion Sickness Remedies

1. Dramamine (see page 124 for more information)
2. Bonine (see page 124 for more information)
3. Dramamine Non-Drowsy Naturals (see page 124 for more information)
4. Sea-Band (see page 124 for more information)
5. Emetrol (see page 124 for more information)
6. Sea-Band Ginger Gum (see page 124 for more information)

Nausea Remedies

1. Dramamine Nausea (see page 124 for more information)
2. Emetrol (see page 124 for more information)
3. Sea-Band (see page 124 for more information)
4. Nauzene (see page 124 for more information)

Proton Pump Inhibitors

1. Prilosec OTC (see page 108 for more information)
2. Nexium 24 HR (see page 107 for more information)
3. Prevacid 24 HR (see page 107 for more information)
4. Zegerid OTC (see page 108 for more information)

Stool Softeners

1. Colace (see pages 118 and 121 for more information)
2. Dulcolax (see pages 118 and 121 for more information)
3. DulcoEase (see page 121 for more information)
4. Phillips' (see pages 119 and 122 for more information)

Upset Stomach Remedies

1. Emetrol (see page 124 for more information)
2. Nauzene (see page 124 for more information)

Ophthalmics and Otics

Artificial Tears / Ophthalmic Lubricants

1. Refresh (see page 129 for more information)
2. Systane (see page 130 for more information)
3. Visine (see page 130 for more information)
4. GenTeal (see page 128 for more information
5. TheraTears (see page 130 for more information)
6. Blink (see page 128 for more information)
7. Advanced Eye Relief (see page 128 for more information)
8. Clear Eyes (see page 128 for more information)

Ophthalmic Antihistamines / Decongestants

1. Systane Zaditor (see page 130 for more information)
2. Pataday (see page 129 for more information)
3. Naphcon-A (see page 129 for more information)
4. Visine (see page 130 for more information)
5. Alaway (see page 128 for more information)
6. Opcon-A (see page 129 for more information)
7. Clear Eyes (see page 128 for more information)

Ear Pain Relief

1. Similasan Earache Relief (see page 139 for more information)
2. Hyland's Earache Drops (see page 139 for more information)
3. TRP Ring Relief (see page 139 for more information)

Ear Wax Removal

1. Debrox (see page 139 for more information)
2. Auro-Dri (see page 139 for more information)
3. NeilMed Clearcanal (see page 139 for more information)
4. Earwax MD (see page 139 for more information)
5. Similasan Ear Wax Relief (see page 139 for more information)

Oral Care

Canker Sore Treatments

1. Orajel (see page 133 for more information)
2. Zilactin-B (see page 133 for more information)
3. Anbesol (see page 131 for more information)
4. Gly-Oxide (see page 132 for more information)
5. Kank-A (see page 132 for more information)
6. DenTek Canker Sore Patch (see page 132 for more information)
7. GUM Canker-X (see page 132 for more information)

Cold Sore Treatments

1. Abreva (see page 131 for more information)
2. Orajel Cold Sore (see page 133 for more information)
3. Carmex Cold Sore Treatment (see page 132 for more information)
4. Lip Clear Lysine (see page 132 for more information)
5. Blister Balm (see page 131 for more information)

Dry Mouth Therapy

1. Biotene (see pages 131 and 134 for more information)
2. OraCoat XyliMelts (see page 133 for more information)
3. GUM Hydral (see page 132 for more information)
4. TheraBreath (see page 133 for more information)
5. ACT Dry Mouth (see pages 131 and 133 for more information)
6. Lubricity (see page 132 for more information)

Mouthwashes / Oral Rinses, Cosmetic

1. Biotene (see page 134 for more information)
2. Scope (see page 135 for more information)
3. Cepacol (see page 134 for more information)
4. Smart Mouth (see page 135 for more information)
5. PLAX (see page 134 for more information)
6. Tom's of Maine (see page 135 for more information)
7. TheraBreath (see page 135 for more information)

Mouthwashes / Oral Rinses, Therapeutic

1. Listerine (see page 134 for more information)
2. Biotene (see page 134 for more information)

3. Crest Pro-Health (see page 134 for more information)
4. Cepacol (see page 134 for more information)
5. CloSYS (see page 134 for more information)
6. TheraBreath (see page 135 for more information)
7. Colgate Phos-Flur (see page 134 for more information)
8. Orajel Antiseptic Rinse (see page 133 for more information)

Oral Pain Relievers, Adult

1. Orajel (see page 133 for more information)
2. Anbesol (see page 131 for more information)
3. Zilactin-B (see page 133 for more information)
4. Benzodent (see page 131 for more information)
5. DenTek (see page 132 for more information)
6. Gly-Oxide (see page 132 for more information)
7. Kank-A (see page 132 for more information)

Sore Throat Products

1. Cepacol (see page 112 for more information)
2. Chloraseptic (lozenges only) (see page 112 for more information)
3. HALLS (see page 112 for more information)
4. Ricola (see page 113 for more information)
5. Fisherman's Friend (see page 112 for more information)
6. Luden's (see page 112 for more information)
7. Sucrets (see page 113 for more information)
8. Zarbee's Honey Cough Soothers (see page 113 for more information)

Toothache Products

1. Orajel (see page 133 for more information)
2. Anbesol (see page 131 for more information)
3. Red Cross Toothache Medication (see page 133 for more information)
4. Kank-A (see page 132 for more information)
5. DenTek (see page 132 for more information)

Toothpaste, General Use

1. Crest (see pages 136 and 137 for more information)
2. Colgate (see page 136 for more information)
3. Sensodyne (see pages 137 and 138 for more information)
4. Parodontax (see page 137 for more information)

5. Arm & Hammer (see page 135 for more information)
6. Aquafresh (see page 135 for more information)
7. Burt's Bees (see page 135 for more information)
8. Tom's of Maine (see page 138 for more information)

Toothpaste, Sensitive Gums / Teeth

1. Sensodyne (see pages 137 and 138 for more information)
2. Crest Sensitive (see page 137 for more information)
3. Colgate Sensitive (see page 136 for more information)
4. Tom's of Maine (see page 138 for more information)
5. Arm & Hammer Sensitive (see page 135 for more information)

Pain and Inflammation

Analgesics, Topical

1. Voltaren Gel (see page 156 for more information)
2. Biofreeze (see page 155 for more information)
3. Aspercreme (see page 155 for more information)
4. Salonpas (see page 156 for more information)
5. BENGAY (see page 155 for more information)
6. Icy Hot (see page 155 for more information)
7. Arnicare (see page 155 for more information)
8. Tiger Balm (see page 156 for more information)
9. Blue Emu (see page 155 for more information)
10. Capzasin-HP (see page 155 for more information)
11. Thera-Gesic (see page 156 for more information)
12. Theraworx Relief (see page 156 for more information)

Analgesics for Arthritis / Joint Pain, Topical

1. Voltaren Gel (see page 156 for more information)
2. Biofreeze (see page 155 for more information)
3. Salonpas (see page 156 for more information)
4. Icy Hot (see page 155 for more information)
5. Aspercreme (see page 155 for more information)
6. BENGAY (see page 155 for more information)
7. Capzasin-HP (see page 155 for more information)
8. Theraworx Relief (see page 156 for more information)
9. Tiger Balm (see page 156 for more information)
10. Thera-Gesic (see page 156 for more information)
11. Australian Dream (see page 155 for more information)

Anti-Inflammatory Products, Oral

1. Advil (see page 101 for more information)
2. Motrin (see page 104 for more information)
3. Aleve (see page 101 for more information)

Arthritis Pain Relievers, Oral

1. Tylenol Arthritis Pain (see page 104 for more information)
2. Advil (see page 101 for more information)

3. Aleve (see page 101 for more information)
4. Motrin (see page 104 for more information)

Headache Products

1. Tylenol (see pages 104 and 105 for more information)
2. Advil (see page 101 for more information)
3. Motrin (see page 104 for more information)
4. Aleve (see page 101 for more information)

Homeopathic Analgesics, Topical

1. Arnicare (see page 155 for more information)
2. Theraworx Relief (see page 156 for more information)
3. Calendula Cream (see page 155 for more information)
4. T-Relief Cream (see page 156 for more information)

Leg Cramp Relief

1. Theraworx Relief (see page 156 for more information)
2. Arnicare Leg Cramps (see page 101 for more information)
3. Legatrin PM (see page 150 for more information)
4. MagniLife Relaxing Legs (see page 103 for more information)
5. Cramp 911 (see page 102 for more information)

Low-Dose Aspirin, Recurrent Heart Attack / Stroke Prevention

1. Bayer (see page 117 for more information)
2. Ecotrin (see page 117 for more information)
3. St. Joseph (see page 117 for more information)

Migraine Headache Products

1. Advil Migraine (see page 101 for more information)
2. Aleve (see page 101 for more information)
3. Tylenol (see pages 104 and 105 for more information)

Thermal Relief Products

1. Salonpas (see page 156 for more information)
2. ThermaCare (see page 156 for more information)
3. Icy Hot Patch (see page 155 for more information)

Sleep Aids

Sleep Aids

1. Unisom SleepGels/SleepMelts (see page 152 for more information)
2. Simply Sleep (see page 151 for more information)
3. Sominex (see page 151 for more information)

Sleep Aids, Alternative

1. Nature Made Melatonin (see page 151 for more information)
2. Natrol Melatonin (see page 151 for more information)
3. Vicks ZzzQuil (see page 152 for more information)
4. Nature's Bounty Melatonin (see page 151 for more information)
5. MidNite (see page 150 for more information)
6. Zarbee's Naturals (see page 152 for more information)

Sleep / Analgesic Combination Products

1. Tylenol PM (see page 152 for more information)
2. Advil PM (see page 150 for more information)
3. Aleve PM (see page 150 for more information)

Smoking Cessation

Smoking Cessation Aids

1. NicoDerm CQ Patch (see page 153 for more information)
2. Nicorette (see page 153 for more information)
3. Habitrol (see page 153 for more information)

Topicals for Skin and Wound Care

Acne Products

1. Differin Gel (see page 87 for more information)
2. Clearasil (see pages 86 and 87 for more information)
3. Neutrogena (see pages 87 and 88 for more information)
4. Cetaphil (see page 86 for more information)
5. PanOxyl (see page 88 for more information)
6. CeraVe (see page 86 for more information)
7. Clean & Clear (see page 86 for more information)
8. OXY (see page 88 for more information)
9. Aveeno (see page 86 for more information)
10. Bioré (see page 86 for more information)
11. Stridex (see page 88 for more information)
12. La Roche-Posay (see page 87 for more information)
13. St. Ives (see page 88 for more information)

Anesthetics, Topical

1. Dermoplast (see page 163 for more information)
2. Bactine (see page 162 for more information)

Antibiotics / Antiseptics, Topical

1. NEOSPORIN (see page 163 for more information)
2. POLYSPORIN (see page 164 for more information)
3. Bacitracin ointment, generic (see page 162 for more information)
4. Bactine (see page 162 for more information)

Antifungal Products, General

1. Lotrimin (see page 157 for more information)
2. Lamisil (see page 157 for more information)
3. Tinactin (see page 158 for more information)
4. Micatin (see page 157 for more information)
5. Zeasorb (see page 158 for more information)

Anti-Itch Products

1. Cortizone-10 (see pages 159 and 160 for more information)
2. Caladryl (see page 159 for more information)

3. Benadryl (Topical) (see page 159 for more information)
4. Aveeno (see page 159 for more information)
5. Domeboro (see page 160 for more information)
6. Gold Bond (see page 160 for more information)
7. Dr. Nice's Moisturizing Gel (see page 160 for more information)

Burn Treatments

1. NEOSPORIN (see page 163 for more information)
2. Dermoplast (see page 163 for more information)
3. A+D Ointment (see page 162 for more information)
4. Alocane (see page 162 for more information)
5. POLYSPORIN (see page 164 for more information)
6. Bacitraycin Plus (see page 162 for more information)
7. Bactine (see page 162 for more information)
8. Foille (see page 163 for more information)
9. Dr. Nice's Moisturizing Gel (see page 163 for more information)

Dandruff Shampoo

1. Head & Shoulders (see pages 114 and 115 for more information)
2. Nizoral (see page 115 for more information)
3. Selsun blue (see pages 115 and 116 for more information)
4. Neutrogena T/Gel (see page 115 for more information)
5. Neutrogena T/Sal (see page 115 for more information)
6. La Roche-Posay Kerium DS (see page 115 for more information)
7. MG217 Psoriasis (see page 115 for more information)

Diabetic Foot Creams

1. Eucerin (see page 142 for more information)
2. CeraVe (see page 141 for more information)
3. Gold Bond (see page 143 for more information)
4. O'Keeffe's for Healthy Feet (see page 145 for more information)
5. Flexitol (see page 143 for more information)
6. Zim's Crack Creme (see page 146 for more information)
7. Kerasal (see page 144 for more information)

Eczema Care / Relief Products

1. CeraVe (see page 159 for more information)
2. Eucerin (see page 160 for more information)

3.   Aquaphor (see page 140 for more information)
4.   Aveeno (see page 159 for more information)
5.   Cetaphil (see page 159 for more information)
6.   Cortizone-10 (see page 160 for more information)
7.   MG217 Eczema (see page 161 for more information)
8.   Gold Bond (see page 160 for more information)
9.   Vanicream (see page 145 for more information)
10. Scalpicin (see pages 115 and 161 for more information)
11. Dr. Nice's Moisturizing Gel (see page 160 for more information)

Foot Care Products

1.   Dr. Scholl's (see pages 111 and 142 for more information)
2.   AmLactin (see page 140 for more information)
3.   Gold Bond (see page 143 for more information)
4.   O'Keefe's for Healthy Feet (see page 145 for more information)
5.   Cetaphil (see pages 141 and 142 for more information)
6.   Kerasal (see page 144 for more information)
7.   Curél (see page 142 for more information)
8.   Odor-Eaters (see page 157 for more information)
9.   Zim's Crack Creme (see page 146 for more information)
10. Duke Cannon Grunt Foot & Boot (see page 142 for more information)

Foot / Toe Antifungal Products (Athlete's Foot, Nail Fungus, etc)

1.   Lamisil (see page 157 for more information)
2.   Lotrimin (see page 157 for more information)
3.   Tinactin (see page 158 for more information)
4.   Fungi-Nail (see page 157 for more information)
5.   Micatin (see page 157 for more information)
6.   Zeasorb (see page 158 for more information)

Hemorrhoidal Preparations

1.   Preparation H (see page 119 for more information)
2.   Tucks (see page 119 for more information)
3.   RectiCare (see page 119 for more information)
4.   Hyland's Hemorrhoids (see page 118 for more information)

Lice Treatments

1.   Nix (see page 148 for more information)

2. RID (see page 148 for more information)
3. Lice MD (see page 148 for more information)
4. Licefreee! (see page 148 for more information)
5. Lice Shield (see page 148 for more information)
6. LiceGuard (see page 148 for more information)

Liquid Bandages

1. New-Skin (see page 164 for more information)
2. Nexcare (see page 164 for more information)
3. Curad FlexSEAL Spray (see page 163 for more information)
4. Dr. Nice's Moisturizing Gel (see page 163 for more information)

Poison Ivy / Oak Remedies

1. Cortizone-10 (see pages 159 and 160 for more information)
2. Caladryl (see page 159 for more information)
3. Ivy-Dry (see pages 160 and 161 for more information)
4. Benadryl (Topical) (see page 159 for more information)
5. Tecnu (see page 161 for more information)
6. Zanfel (see page 161 for more information)
7. Aveeno (see page 159 for more information)
8. Ivarest (see page 160 for more information)
9. Domeboro (see page 160 for more information)
10. Gold Bond (see page 160 for more information)
11. Sarna (see page 161 for more information)

Scar Treatments

1. Mederma (see pages 144 and 146 for more information)
2. Bio-Oil (see page 141 for more information)
3. Palmer's Skin Therapy Oil (see page 145 for more information)
4. ScarAway (see page 147 for more information)
5. Cicatricure (see page 146 for more information)
6. Scarguard (see page 147 for more information)

Stretch Mark Treatments

1. Mederma Stretch Marks Therapy (see page 146 for more information)
2. Palmer's Stretch Marks (see page 147 for more information)
3. Bio-Oil (see page 141 for more information)
4. SheaMoisture (see page 145 for more information)

5. Mustela (see page 146 for more information)
6. Queen Helene Cocoa Butter Crème (see page 145 for more information)

Sunburn Relief

1. Dermoplast (see page 163 for more information)
2. Banana Boat (see page 141 for more information)
3. Alocane (see page 162 for more information)
4. Hawaiian Tropic (see page 143 for more information)
5. SunBurnt (see page 145 for more information)
6. Australian Gold (see page 141 for more information)
7. Dr. Nice Moisturizing Gel (see page 163 for more information)

Sunscreens (see pages 55 and 56 for more information)

1. Neutrogena
2. Coppertone
3. Banana Boat
4. Blue Lizard
5. Bullfrog
6. CeraVe
7. Hawaiian Tropic
8. La Roche-Posay
9. Aveeno
10. Australian Gold
11. Sun Bum
12. Vanicream
13. Baby Bum
14. Babyganics
15. Panama Jack

Therapeutic Skin Care, Cleansers

1. Cetaphil (see page 86 for more information)
2. CeraVe (see page 86 for more information)
3. Aveeno (see page 86 for more information)
4. Eucerin (see page 87 for more information)
5. Neutrogena (see pages 87 and 88 for more information)
6. Dove (see page 87 for more information)
7. Clean & Clear (see page 86 for more information)
8. Olay (see page 88 for more information)
9. Vanicream (see page 88 for more information)

Therapeutic Skin Care, Moisturizers

1. CeraVe (see page 141 for more information)
2. Eucerin (see pages 142 and 143 for more information)
3. Aquaphor (see page 140 for more information)
4. AmLactin (see page 140 for more information)
5. Cetaphil (see pages 141 and 142 for more information)
6. Aveeno (see page 141 for more information)
7. Gold Bond (see page 143 for more information)
8. Lubriderm (see page 144 for more information)
9. Vaseline (see page 146 for more information)
10. Curél (see page 142 for more information)
11. Jergens (see pages 143 and 144 for more information)
12. Palmer's Cocoa Butter Formula (see page 145 for more information)
13. Vanicream (see page 145 for more information)
14. O'Keeffe's Working Hands (see page 145 for more information)
15. Neutrogena (see page 144 for more information)
16. Nivea (see page 145 for more information)
17. Dr. Nice's Moisturizing Gel (see page 142 for more information)

Wart Removers

1. Compound W (see page 111 for more information)
2. Dr. Scholl's Freeze Away (see page 111 for more information)
3. Curad Mediplast (see page 111 for more information)
4. WartStick (see page 111 for more information)
5. ProVent Wart Remover (see page 111 for more information)
6. Wartner (see page 111 for more information)

Women's Health

Urinary Health
1. AZO Urinary Pain Relief (see page 102 for more information)
2. Uristat (see page 105 for more information)

Yeast Infection Prevention and Relief
1. MONISTAT (see page 165 for more information)
2. AZO Yeast Plus (see page 165 for more information)
3. Florajen (see page 165 for more information)
4. Vagisil (see page 166 for more information)
5. RepHresh Pro-B (see page 165 for more information)
6. Cortizone-10 Feminine Itch (see page 165 for more information)
7. Jarro-Dophilus Women (see page 165 for more information)
8. Vagistat (see page 166 for more information)
9. YeastGard (see page 166 for more information)

Vaginal Moisturizers and Lubricants
1. K-Y (see page 165 for more information)
2. Replens (see page 165 for more information)
3. Vagisil Lubricant (see page 166 for more information)
4. Astroglide (see page 165 for more information)
5. Lubrigyn (see page 165 for more information)
6. Damiva (see page 165 for more information)
7. Luvena (see page 165 for more information)

5.
OVER-THE-COUNTER PRODUCTS

What Is Covered In These Tables?

In this section, you will find comprehensive tables describing the safety levels of specific and generic OTC products available in the United States. There are over 300,000 nonprescription products available today, and it is not possible to list every available preparation. In this work, approximately 1,700 nonprescription preparations have been chosen to best represent those that someone who is breastfeeding might wish to use.

In addition, each product in each table lists the active or relevant ingredients in alphabetical order.

Pediatric (children's) or men's health OTC preparations are not included in the tables, as most breastfeeding parents would not be taking these medications to treat themselves.

If a specific OTC product that you are looking for is not listed, check the corresponding active ingredients table to determine if the medication is compatible with breastfeeding. If there is any doubt, it is best to consult with your doctor or pharmacist.

Directory of OTC Product Tables

Acne Products and Facial Cleansers

		SAFETY LEVEL (PAGE 19)	DO NOT APPLY TO BREASTS
Aveeno Calm + Restore Gentle Nourishing Oat Face Cleanser *(feverfew / oat kernel flour / poloxamer 188)*	OK	L1	
Aveeno Clear Complexion Bar / Clear Complexion Foaming Cleanser *(salicylic acid)*	OK	L2	*
Aveeno Positively Radiant Skin Brightening Face Cleanser *(cocamidopropyl betaine / soy extract)*	OK	L1	
Aveeno Ultra-Calming Foaming Cleanser *(cocamidopropyl betaine / feverfew)*	OK	L1	
Benzoyl peroxide bar / cleanser / cream / gel / wash, generic *(benzoyl peroxide)*	OK	L1	*
Bioré Blemish Fighting Ice Cleanser *(salicylic acid)*	OK	L2	*
CeraVe Acne Control Cleanser *(salicylic acid)*	OK	L2	*
CeraVe Acne Foaming Cream Cleanser *(benzoyl peroxide)*	OK	L1	*
CeraVe Hydrating Facial Cleanser *(ceramides / cetearyl alcohol / hyaluronic acid)*	OK	L1	
CeraVe Renewing SA Cleanser *(salicylic acid)*	OK	L2	*
Cetaphil Daily Facial Cleanser *(cocamidopropyl betaine)*	OK	L1	
Cetaphil DermaControl Oil Removing Foam Wash *(zinc coceth sulfate)*	OK	L1	
Cetaphil Gentle Clear Clarifying Acne Cream Cleanser *(salicylic acid)*	OK	L2	*
Clean & Clear Advantage Acne Spot Treatment / Advantage Oil-Free Acne Moisturizer *(salicylic acid)*	OK	L1	*
Clean & Clear Blackhead Clearing Daily Cleansing Pads / Blackhead Cleansing Scrub *(salicylic acid)*	OK	L2	*
Clean & Clear Continuous Control Acne Wash Oil-Free *(salicylic acid)*	OK	L2	*
Clean & Clear Morning Burst Cleanser *(citrus extracts / cocamidopropyl betaine / ginseng)*	OK	L1	*
Clearasil Acne Treatment Tinted Cream *(benzoyl peroxide)*	OK	L1	*

Product		Safety Level (Page 19)	Do Not Apply to Breasts
Clearasil Stay Clear Acne Fighting Cleansing Wipes / Stay Clear Daily Facial Scrub / Stay Clear Daily Pore Cleansing Pads / Stay Clear Oil-Free Gel Wash / Stay Clear Skin Perfecting Wash *(salicylic acid)*	OK	L2	*
Clearasil Stay Clear Vanishing Acne Treatment Cream *(benzoyl peroxide)*	OK	L2	*
Clearasil Total Acne Control *(benzoyl peroxide)*	OK	L1	*
Clearasil Ultra Acne Clearing Gel Wash / Ultra Daily Face Wash / Ultra Deep Pore Cleansing Pads *(salicylic acid)*	OK	L2	*
Clearasil Ultra Acne Rapid Action Treatment Vanishing Cream *(benzoyl peroxide)*	OK	L1	*
Differin Gel *(adapalene)*	OK	L3	*
Dove Deep Pure Face Cleanser *(lauramidopropyl betaine)*	OK	L1	
Eucerin Gentle Hydrating Foaming Cleanser *(cocamidopropyl betaine / lanolin alcohol / urea)*	OK	L1	
Eucerin Redness Relief Cleansing Gel *(glyceryl cocoate / glycyrrhiza inflata)*	OK	L1	
La Roche-Posay Effaclar Medicated Acne Face Wash *(salicylic acid)*	OK	L2	*
Neutrogena Acne Stress Control 3-in-1 Hydrating Acne Treatment / Oil-Free Acne Stress Control Power Clear Scrub *(salicylic acid)*	OK	L2	*
Neutrogena Advanced Solutions Acne Mark Fading Peel with CelluZyme *(salicylic acid)*	OK	L2	*
Neutrogena Blackhead Eliminating Daily Scrub / Blackhead Eliminating Foaming Pads *(salicylic acid)*	OK	L2	*
Neutrogena Body Clear Body Scrub *(salicylic acid)*	OK	L2	*
Neutrogena Clear Pore Cleanser Mask *(benzoyl peroxide)*	OK	L1	*
Neutrogena Clear Pore Oil-Eliminating Astringent *(salicylic acid)*	OK	L2	*
Neutrogena Oil-Free Acne Wash Cleansing Cloths / Oil-Free Acne Wash Cream Cleanser / Oil-Free Acne Wash Foam Cleanser / Oil-Free Anti-Acne Moisturizer *(salicylic acid)*	OK	L2	*
Neutrogena On-the-Spot Acne Treatment Vanishing Formula *(benzoyl peroxide)*	OK	L1	*

* *Additional note applies*   87   OK *OK to use*   UNSAFE *Do not use*

		SAFETY LEVEL (PAGE 19)	DO NOT APPLY TO BREASTS
Neutrogena Rapid Clear Acne Defense Face Lotion *(salicylic acid)*	OK	L2	✳
Neutrogena Triple Clean Anti-Blemish Astringent / Triple Clean Anti-Blemish Pads *(salicylic acid)*	OK	L2	✳
Neutrogena Ultra Gentle Daily Cleanser *(cocamidopropyl betaine / glycerin)*	OK	L1	
Noxzema Triple Clean Anti-Bacterial Lathering Cleanser *(triclosan)*	OK	L1	✳
Olay Clarifying Daily Facial Cleanser *(salicylic acid)*	OK	L2	✳
Olay Regenerist Regenerating Cream Cleanser *(salicylic acid)*	OK	L2	✳
OXY Advanced Care Maximum Strength Rapid Spot Treatment / Advanced Care Maximum Strength Soothing Cream Acne Cleanser *(benzoyl peroxide)*	OK	L1	✳
OXY Daily Defense Deep Pore Cleansing Pads *(salicylic acid)*	OK	L2	✳
OXY Maximum Strength 3-in-1 Acne Pads *(salicylic acid)*	OK	L2	✳
PanOxyl Acne Creamy Wash Benzoyl Peroxide 4% Daily Control / Acne Foaming Wash Benzoyl Peroxide 10% Maximum Strength *(benzoyl peroxide)*	OK	L1	✳
pHisoderm Anti-Blemish Body Wash / Gel Cleanser *(salicylic acid)*	OK	L2	✳
St. Ives Acne Control Apricot Face Scrub *(salicylic acid)*	OK	L2	✳
Stridex Essential Pads / Maximum Pads / Sensitive Pads *(salicylic acid)*	OK	L2	✳
Vanicream Gentle Facial Cleanser *(coco glucoside / sodium cocoyl glycinate)*	OK	L1	
ZAPZYT Acne Treatment Gel *(benzoyl peroxide)*	OK	L1	✳
ZAPZYT Acne Wash Cleanser *(salicylic acid)*	OK	L2	✳

Allergy, Cold, and Flu Products

A note about pseudoephedrine:

Federal regulation has made it so **PSEUDOEPHEDRINE** (the active ingredient in Sudafed) is kept behind the counter in drugstores and grocery stores. You will not find products containing pseudoephedrine on the shelves, but anyone over the age of 18 can still purchase them without a prescription at the pharmacy counter. You will be required to present a photo ID or provide personal information. Check your state laws for additional restrictions.

Occasional or short-term use of pseudoephedrine is compatible with early stage breastfeeding for parents with good milk production. **Avoid use if poor milk supply is a concern**, especially after six months postpartum.

Because of the regulations, some manufacturers have substituted **PHENYLEPHRINE** for pseudoephedrine. Check labels carefully.

	SAFETY LEVEL (P. 19)	MONITOR INFANT FOR DROWS-INESS	MONITOR MILK SUPPLY & DRINK EXTRA FLUIDS	LOOK FOR ALTERNATIVE THAT DOES NOT COMBINE INGREDIENTS	LOOK FOR ALTERNATIVE THAT IS NOT LONG-ACTING
Advil Allergy & Congestion Relief Coated Tablets / Multi-Symptom Cold & Flu Coated Tablets *(chlorpheniramine / ibuprofen / phenylephrine)*	OK L3	✳	✳	✳	
Advil Allergy Sinus Caplets *(chlorpheniramine / ibuprofen / pseudoephedrine)*	OK L3	✳	✳	✳	
Advil Cold & Sinus Caplets / Cold & Sinus Liqui-Gels *(ibuprofen / pseudoephedrine)*	OK L3		✳	✳	
Advil Sinus Congestion & Pain Coated Tablets *(ibuprofen / phenylephrine)*	OK L3		✳	✳	
Airborne Dual Action Tablets *(minerals / multivitamins)*	OK L1				

	SAFETY LEVEL (P. 19)	MONITOR INFANT FOR DROWS-INESS	MONITOR MILK SUPPLY & DRINK EXTRA FLUIDS	LOOK FOR ALTERNATIVE THAT DOES NOT COMBINE INGREDIENTS	LOOK FOR ALTERNATIVE THAT IS NOT LONG-ACTING
Alavert 24 Hour Allergy Orally Disintegrating Tablets (loratadine)	OK L1	✳			✳
Alavert D-12 Hour Allergy and Congestion Tablets (loratadine / pseudoephedrine)	OK L3	✳	✳	✳	✳
Aleve-D Cold & Sinus Caplets / Sinus & Headache Caplets (naproxen / pseudoephedrine)	OK L3		✳	✳	
Alka-Seltzer Plus Cold & Cough Liquid Gels / Plus Cold & Cough PowerMax Gels (acetaminophen / chlorpheniramine / dextromethorphan / phenylephrine)	OK L3	✳	✳	✳	
Alka-Seltzer Plus Cold & Flu Effervescent Tablets / Plus Sinus Congestion & Pain Effervescent Tablets (acetaminophen / chlorpheniramine / dextromethorphan / phenylephrine)	OK L3	✳	✳	✳	
Alka-Seltzer Plus Cold Non-Drowsy Effervescent Tablets (aspirin / dextromethorphan / phenylephrine)	UNSAFE L4				
Alka-Seltzer Plus Cold Original Effervescent Tablets (aspirin / chlorpheniramine / phenylephrine)	UNSAFE L4				
Alka-Seltzer Plus Cough & Chest Congestion Effervescent Tablets (dextromethorphan / guaifenesin)	OK L2	✳		✳	
Alka-Seltzer Plus Day Cold & Flu Mix-In Powder (acetaminophen / dextromethorphan / guaifenesin / phenylephrine)	OK L3	✳	✳	✳	
Alka-Seltzer Plus Day Cold & Flu PowerMax Gels (acetaminophen / dextromethorphan / phenylephrine)	OK L3	✳	✳	✳	
Alka-Seltzer Plus Night Cold & Flu Mix-In Powder / Plus Night Cold & Flu PowerMax Gels (acetaminophen / dextromethorphan / doxylamine / phenylephrine)	OK L3	✳	✳	✳	

OK *OK to use*   UNSAFE *Do not use*   90   ✳ *Additional note applies*

	SAFETY LEVEL (P. 19)	MONITOR INFANT FOR DROWS-INESS	MONITOR MILK SUPPLY & DRINK EXTRA FLUIDS	LOOK FOR ALTERNATIVE THAT DOES NOT COMBINE INGREDIENTS	LOOK FOR ALTERNATIVE THAT IS NOT LONG-ACTING
Alka-Seltzer Plus Night Cold Effervescent Tablets *(aspirin / dextromethorphan / doxylamine / phenylephrine)*	UNSAFE	L4				
Allegra Allergy 12 Hour Tablets / 24 Hour Gelcaps / 24 Hour Tablets *(fexofenadine)*	OK	L2	*	*		*
Allegra-D 12 Hour Allergy & Congestion Tablets / 24 Hour Allergy & Congestion Tablets *(fexofenadine / pseudoephedrine)*	OK	L3	*	*	*	*
Allerest Maximum Strength Tablets *(chlorpheniramine / pseudoephedrine)*	OK	L3	*	*	*	
Allerest No Drowsiness Allergy & Sinus Caplets *(acetaminophen / pseudoephedrine)*	OK	L3		*	*	
Allerest PE Allergy & Sinus Relief Tablets *(chlorpheniramine / phenylephrine*	OK	L3	*	*	*	
Benadryl Allergy Extra Strength Ultratabs / Allergy Liqui-Gels / Allergy Ultratabs *(diphenhydramine)*	OK	L2	*	*		
Benadryl Allergy Plus Congestion *(diphenhydramine / phenylephrine)*	OK	L3	*	*	*	
Benylin All-In-One Cold & Flu Night Syrup *(acetaminophen / chlorpheniramine / dextromethorphan / guaifenesin / pseudoephedrine)*	OK	L3	*	*	*	
Benylin All-In-One Cold & Flu Syrup / Cold & Sinus Liquid Gels *(acetaminophen / dextromethorphan / guaifenesin / pseudoephedrine)*	OK	L3	*	*	*	
Benylin Chest Congestion & Cold Syrup *(guaifenesin / menthol)*	OK	L2	*		*	
Benylin Chesty Coughs Non-Drowsy Syrup *(guaifenesin)*	OK	L2				

	SAFETY LEVEL (P. 19)	MONITOR INFANT FOR DROWS- INESS	MONITOR MILK SUPPLY & DRINK EXTRA FLUIDS	LOOK FOR ALTERNATIVE THAT DOES NOT COMBINE INGREDIENTS	LOOK FOR ALTERNATIVE THAT IS NOT LONG- ACTING
Benylin Cough & Chest Congestion Syrup / Extra Strength Cough & Chest Congestion Syrup *(dextromethorphan / guaifenesin)*	OK L2	✳		✳	
Benylin Cough Complete Syrup *(dextromethorphan / guaifenesin / menthol / pseudoephedrine)*	OK L3	✳	✳	✳	
Benylin Dry Cough Syrup *(dextromethorphan)*	OK L1	✳			
Benylin Mucus Cough Max Menthol Syrup *(menthol)*	OK L2				
Boiron Chestal Cough and Cold Syrup *(homeopathic herbs)*	OK L3	✳			
Boiron ColdCalm Tablets *(homeopathic herbs)*	UNSAFE L4				
Boiron Oscillococcinum Pellets *(Anas barbariae)*	UNSAFE L4				
Claritin 24 Hour Allergy Tablets *(loratadine)*	OK L1	✳			✳
Claritin-D 12 Hour Allergy & Congestion Tablets *(loratadine / pseudoephedrine)*	OK L1	✳	✳	✳	✳
Claritin-D 24 Hour Allergy & Congestion Tablets *(loratadine / pseudoephedrine)*	OK L1	✳	✳	✳	✳
Cold-EEZE Plus Defense Chewable Gels *(zinc gluconate)*	OK L1				
Contac Cold & Flu Day Caplets *(acetaminophen / phenylephrine)*	OK L3		✳	✳	
Contac Cold & Flu Night Caplets *(acetaminophen / chlorpheniramine / phenylephrine)*	OK L3	✳	✳	✳	
Contac Cold & Flu Night Cooling Relief Liquid *(acetaminophen / dextromethorphan / doxylamine)*	OK L3	✳	✳	✳	

	SAFETY LEVEL (P. 19)	MONITOR INFANT FOR DROWS-INESS	MONITOR MILK SUPPLY & DRINK EXTRA FLUIDS	LOOK FOR ALTERNATIVE THAT DOES NOT COMBINE INGREDIENTS	LOOK FOR ALTERNATIVE THAT IS NOT LONG-ACTING
Coricidin HBP Chest Congestion & Cough Liquid Gels *(dextromethorphan / guaifenesin)*	OK L2	*		*	
Coricidin HBP Cold & Flu Tablets *(acetaminophen / chlorpheniramine)*	OK L3	*	*	*	
Coricidin HBP Cough & Cold Tablets *(chlorpheniramine / dextromethorphan)*	OK L3	*	*	*	
Coricidin HBP Maximum Strength Cold, Flu, & Chest Congestion Liquid Gels *(acetaminophen / guaifenesin)*	OK L2			*	
Coricidin HBP Maximum Strength Multi-Symptom Flu Tablets *(acetaminophen / chlorpheniramine / dextromethorphan)*	OK L3	*	*	*	
Coricidin HBP Maximum Strength Nighttime Cold & Flu Liquid *(acetaminophen / dextromethorphan / doxylamine)*	OK L3	*	*	*	
CVS Health 4-Hour Allergy Relief Tablets *(chlorpheniramine)*	OK L3	*	*		
DayClear Cough Cold & Flu Relief Liquid *(choline salicylate / dextromethorphan / guaifenesin / phenylephrine)*	UNSAFE L4				
Delsym 12 Hour Cough Relief Suspension *(dextromethorphan)*	OK L1	*			*
Delsym Nighttime Cough Fast Release Suspension *(acetaminophen / dextromethorphan / triprolidine)*	OK L3	*	*	*	
Diabetic Tussin Chest Congestion *(guaifenesin)*	OK L2				
Diabetic Tussin Cough & Chest Congestion DM *(dextromethorphan / guaifenesin)*	OK L3	*	*	*	

* *Additional note applies*　　　93　　　OK *OK to use*　　UNSAFE *Do not use*

	SAFETY LEVEL (P. 19)	MONITOR INFANT FOR DROWS-INESS	MONITOR MILK SUPPLY & DRINK EXTRA FLUIDS	LOOK FOR ALTERNATIVE THAT DOES NOT COMBINE INGREDIENTS	LOOK FOR ALTERNATIVE THAT IS NOT LONG-ACTING
Diabetic Tussin Nighttime Cold & Flu Suspension *(acetaminophen / dextromethorphan / diphenhydramine)*	OK L3	*	*	*	
Dristan Cold Multi-Symptom Tablets *(acetaminophen / chlorpheniramine / phenylephrine)*	OK L3	*	*	*	
Hyland's Defend Cough + Mucus Syrup *(homeopathic herbs)*	UNSAFE L4				
Hyland's Defend Cough Syrup *(homeopathic herbs)*	UNSAFE L4				
Mucinex D Maximum Strength Expectorant and Nasal Decongestant Tablets *(guaifenesin / pseudoephedrine)*	OK L3		*	*	
Mucinex DM Extended-Release Bi-Layer Tablets *(dextromethorphan / guaifenesin)*	OK L2	*	*		*
Mucinex Extended-Release Bi-Layer Tablets *(guaifenesin)*	OK L2				*
Mucinex Sinus-Max Pressure, Pain & Cough Caplets / Sinus-Max Pressure, Pain & Cough Liquid Gels *(acetaminophen / dextromethorphan / guaifenesin / phenylephrine)*	OK L3	*	*	*	
Nexafed Nasal Decongestant Tablets *(pseudoephedrine)*	OK L3		*		
Nexafed Sinus Pressure + Pain Tablets *(acetaminophen / pseudoephedrine)*	OK L3		*	*	
Refenesen Chest Congestion Relief Caplets *(guaifenesin)*	OK L2				
Robitussin Cough & Chest Congestion DM Liquid / Cough & Chest Congestion DM Liquid Capsules / Sugar-Free Cough & Chest Congestion DM Liquid *(dextromethorphan / guaifenesin)*	OK L2	*		*	

OK *OK to use*   UNSAFE *Do not use*   * *Additional note applies*

		SAFETY LEVEL (P. 19)	MONITOR INFANT FOR DROWS- INESS	MONITOR MILK SUPPLY & DRINK EXTRA FLUIDS	LOOK FOR ALTERNATIVE THAT DOES NOT COMBINE INGREDIENTS	LOOK FOR ALTERNATIVE THAT IS NOT LONG- ACTING
Robitussin 12 Hour Cough Relief Liquid / Long-Acting CoughGels *(dextromethorphan)*	OK	L1	*		*	*
Robitussin Multi-Symptom Cold CF Liquid *(dextromethorphan / guaifenesin / phenylephrine)*	OK	L3	*	*	*	
Robitussin Nighttime Cough DM Liquid *(dextromethorphan / doxylamine)*	OK	L3	*	*	*	
Robitussin Nighttime Severe Multi-Symptom Cough, Cold + Flu CF Liquid *(acetaminophen / diphenhydramine / phenylephrine)*	OK	L3	*	*	*	
Robitussin Severe Cough + Sore Throat CF Liquid *(acetaminophen / dextromethorphan)*	OK	L2	*		*	
Robitussin Severe Multi-Symptom Cough, Cold + Flu CF Liquid *(acetaminophen / dextromethorphan / guaifenesin / phenylephrine)*	OK	L3	*	*	*	
Safetussin DM Daytime Cough Relief Liquid *(dextromethorphan / guaifenesin)*	OK	L2	*		*	
Safetussin PM Nighttime Cough Relief Liquid *(dextromethorphan / doxylamine)*	OK	L3	*	*	*	
Sambucol Black Elderberry Cold & Flu Relief Tablets *(elderberry / homeopathic herbs)*	OK	L3	*			
Sambucol Black Elderberry Syrup *(elderberry)*	OK	L1				
Scot-Tussin Diabetes CF Sugar-Free Liquid *(dextromethorphan)*	OK	L1	*			
Scot-Tussin DM *(chlorpheniramine / dextromethorphan)*	OK	L3	*	*	*	
Scot-Tussin DM Maximum Strength Sugar-Free Liquid *(chlorpheniramine / dextromethorphan)*	OK	L3	*	*	*	

* *Additional note applies*   OK *OK to use*   UNSAFE *Do not use*

		SAFETY LEVEL (P. 19)	MONITOR INFANT FOR DROWS-INESS	MONITOR MILK SUPPLY & DRINK EXTRA FLUIDS	LOOK FOR ALTERNATIVE THAT DOES NOT COMBINE INGREDIENTS	LOOK FOR ALTERNATIVE THAT IS NOT LONG-ACTING
Scot-Tussin Senior Sugar-Free Liquid *(dextromethorphan / guaifenesin)*	OK	L2	*	*	*	
Silphen Cough Syrup *(diphenhydramine)*	OK	L2	*	*		
Silphen Cough Syrup DM *(dextromethorphan)*	OK	L1	*			
Sinarest Drops *(acetaminophen / chlorpheniramine / phenylephrine)*	OK	L3	*	*	*	
Sinarest Syrup *(acetaminophen / chlorpheniramine / phenylephrine / sodium citrate)*	OK	L3	*	*	*	
Sinarest Tablets *(acetaminophen / caffeine / chlorpheniramine)*	OK	L3	*	*	*	
Sine-Off Multi-Symptom Relief Severe Cold Medicine Tablets *(acetaminophen / guaifenesin / phenylephrine)*	OK	L3		*	*	
Sine-Off Non-Drowsy Relief Maximum Strength Caplets *(acetaminophen / phenylephrine)*	OK	L3		*	*	
Sinutab Sinus Caplets *(acetaminophen / phenylephrine)*	OK	L3		*	*	
Sudafed PE Head Congestion + Mucus Tablets *(acetaminophen / guaifenesin / phenylephrine)*	OK	L3		*	*	
Sudafed PE Head Congestion + Pain Tablets *(ibuprofen / phenylephrine)*	OK	L3		*	*	
Sudafed PE Nighttime Sinus Congestion Tablets *(diphenhydramine / phenylephrine)*	OK	L3	*	*	*	
Sudafed PE Sinus Congestion Tablets *(phenylephrine)*	OK	L3		*		
Sudafed PE Sinus Pressure + Pain Tablets *(acetaminophen / phenylephrine)*	OK	L3		*	*	

	SAFETY LEVEL (P. 19)	MONITOR INFANT FOR DROWS-INESS	MONITOR MILK SUPPLY & DRINK EXTRA FLUIDS	LOOK FOR ALTERNATIVE THAT DOES NOT COMBINE INGREDIENTS	LOOK FOR ALTERNATIVE THAT IS NOT LONG-ACTING
Sudafed Sinus 12 Hour Pressure + Pain Tablets *(naproxen / pseudoephedrine)*	OK L3		✳	✳	✳
Sudafed Sinus Congestion 12 Hour Tablets / Sinus Congestion 24 Hour Tablets *(pseudoephedrine)*	OK L3		✳		✳
Sudafed Sinus Congestion Tablets *(pseudoephedrine)*	OK L3		✳		
Theraflu Daytime Flu Relief Max Strength Hot Liquid Powder / Daytime Flu Relief Max Strength Syrup *(acetaminophen / dextromethorphan)*	OK L3	✳	✳	✳	
Theraflu ExpressMax Daytime Severe Cold & Cough Caplets / ExpressMax Severe Cold & Cough Syrup / Multi-Symptom Severe Cold Hot Liquid Powder / Severe Cold & Cough Hot Liquid Powder *(acetaminophen / dextromethorphan / phenylephrine)*	OK L3	✳	✳	✳	
Theraflu ExpressMax Nighttime Severe Cold & Cough Caplets / ExpressMax Nighttime Severe Cold & Cough Syrup / Nighttime Severe Cold & Cough Hot Liquid Powder *(acetaminophen / diphenhydramine / phenylephrine)*	OK L3	✳	✳	✳	
Theraflu Nighttime Flu Relief Max Strength Hot Liquid Powder / Nighttime Flu Relief Max Strength Syrup *(acetaminophen / chlorpheniramine / dextromethorphan)*	OK L3	✳	✳	✳	
Tylenol Cold Max Caplets *(acetaminophen / dextromethorphan / phenylephrine)*	OK L3	✳	✳	✳	

	SAFETY LEVEL (P. 19)	MONITOR INFANT FOR DROWS-INESS	MONITOR MILK SUPPLY & DRINK EXTRA FLUIDS	LOOK FOR ALTERNATIVE THAT DOES NOT COMBINE INGREDIENTS	LOOK FOR ALTERNATIVE THAT IS NOT LONG-ACTING
Tylenol Cold + Flu Severe Caplets / Cold + Flu Severe Honey Lemon Warming Liquid / Cold + Mucus Severe Cool Burst Liquid *(acetaminophen / dextromethorphan / guaifenesin / phenylephrine)*	OK L3	✳	✳	✳	
Tylenol Extra Strength Cold + Flu Multi-Action Daytime Pain Relief Caplets *(acetaminophen / dextromethorphan / pseudoephedrine)*	OK L3	✳	✳	✳	
Tylenol Extra Strength Cold + Flu Multi-Action Nighttime Pain Relief Caplets *(acetaminophen / chlorpheniramine / dextromethorphan / pseudoephedrine)*	OK L3	✳	✳	✳	
Tylenol For Children & Adults Dye-Free Pain + Fever Liquid *(acetaminophen)*	OK L1				
Tylenol Nighttime Cold + Flu + Cough Wild Berry Burst Liquid *(acetaminophen / dextromethorphan / doxylamine / phenylephrine)*	OK L3	✳	✳	✳	
Tylenol Nighttime Cold + Flu Severe Caplets *(acetaminophen / chlorpheniramine / dextromethorphan / phenylephrine)*	OK L3	✳	✳	✳	
Tylenol Sinus + Headache Non-Drowsy Caplets *(acetaminophen / phenylephrine)*	OK L3		✳	✳	
Tylenol Sinus Severe Pain Relief Caplets *(acetaminophen / guaifenesin / phenylephrine)*	OK L3		✳	✳	
Umcka Cold + Flu Chewables / Cold + Flu Syrup *(homeopathic herbs)*	OK L3				
Umcka ColdCare Chewables / ColdCare Drops / ColdCare Soothing Hot Drink / ColdCare Syrup *(homeopathic herbs)*	OK L3				

	SAFETY LEVEL (P. 19)	MONITOR INFANT FOR DROWS- INESS	MONITOR MILK SUPPLY & DRINK EXTRA FLUIDS	LOOK FOR ALTERNATIVE THAT DOES NOT COMBINE INGREDIENTS	LOOK FOR ALTERNATIVE THAT IS NOT LONG- ACTING
Vicks DayQuil Cold & Flu Relief Liquicaps / DayQuil Cold & Flu Relief Liquid (acetaminophen / dextromethorphan / phenylephrine)	OK L3	*	*	*	
Vicks DayQuil Cough DM + Congestion Relief Liquid (dextromethorphan / guaifenesin / phenylephrine)	OK L3	*	*	*	
Vicks DayQuil Severe Cold & Flu Relief LiquiCaps / DayQuil Severe Cold & Flu Relief Liquid / DayQuil VapoCool Severe Cold & Flu + Congestion Relief Caplets / DayQuil VapoCool Severe Cold & Flu + Congestion Relief Liquid (acetaminophen / dextromethorphan / guaifenesin / phenylephrine)	OK L3	*	*	*	
Vicks Jarabe Cough + Congestion Relief Liquid (dextromethorphan / guaifenesin)	OK L2	*		*	
Vicks NyQuil Alcohol-Free Cold & Flu Relief Liquid (acetaminophen / chlorpheniramine / dextromethorphan)	OK L3	*	*	*	
Vicks NyQuil Cold & Flu Relief Liquicaps / NyQuil Cold & Flu Relief Liquid (acetaminophen / dextromethorphan / doxylamine)	OK L3	*	*	*	
Vicks NyQuil Cough DM + Congestion Relief Liquid (dextromethorphan / doxylamine / phenylephrine)	OK L3	*	*	*	
Vicks NyQuil Severe Cold & Flu Relief LiquiCaps / NyQuil Severe Cold & Flu Relief Liquid (acetaminophen / dextromethorphan / doxylamine / phenylephrine)	OK L3	*	*	*	

* Additional note applies   99   OK OK to use   UNSAFE Do not use

	SAFETY LEVEL (P. 19)	MONITOR INFANT FOR DROWS- INESS	MONITOR MILK SUPPLY & DRINK EXTRA FLUIDS	LOOK FOR ALTERNATIVE THAT DOES NOT COMBINE INGREDIENTS	LOOK FOR ALTERNATIVE THAT IS NOT LONG- ACTING
Vicks NyQuil VapoCool Severe Cold & Flu + Congestion Relief Caplets / NyQuil VapoCool Severe Cold & Flu + Congestion Relief Liquid *(acetaminophen / dextromethorphan / doxylamine / phenylephrine)*	OK L3	*	*	*	
Vicks Sinex Severe All In One Sinus LiquiCaps *(acetaminophen / phenylephrine)*	OK L3		*	*	
Vicks Sinex Severe All In One Sinus + Mucus LiquiCaps *(acetaminophen / guaifenesin / phenylephrine)*	OK L3		*	*	
Wal-Act D Tablets *(pseudoephedrine / tripolidine)*	OK L3	*	*	*	
Zephrex-D Softgels *(pseudoephedrine)*	OK L3		*		
Zicam Cold Remedy RapidMelts / Cold Remedy Ultra RapidMelts *(zinc)*	OK L1				
Zyrtec Tablets *(cetirizine)*	OK L2	*			
Zyrtec-D Tablets *(cetirizine / pseudoephedrine)*	OK L3	*	*	*	

Analgesics (Pain Relievers) and Antipyretics (Fever Reducers)

	SAFETY LEVEL (P. 19)		MONITOR INFANT FOR DROWSINESS OR EXCITABILITY	LOOK FOR ALTERNATIVE THAT DOES NOT COMBINE INGREDIENTS	MONITOR MILK SUPPLY & DRINK EXTRA FLUIDS
Acetaminophen tablets, generic *(acetaminophen)*	OK	L1			
Actidose with Sorbitol Suspension *(activated charcoal / sorbitol)*	OK	L1			
Actidose-Aqua Suspension *(activated charcoal)*	OK	L1			
Advil Caplets / Gel Caplets / Liqui-Gels / Migraine Capsules / Tablets *(ibuprofen)*	OK	L1			
Aleve Caplets / Liquid Gels / Smooth Gels *(naproxen)*	OK	L3			
Alka-Seltzer Extra Strength Effervescent Tablets / Original Effervescent Tablets *(aspirin / sodium bicarbonate)*	UNSAFE	L4			
Alka-Seltzer Hangover Relief Effervescent Tablets *(aspirin / caffeine)*	UNSAFE	L4			
Anacin Advanced Headache Tablets *(acetaminophen / aspirin / caffeine)*	UNSAFE	L4			
Anacin Aspirin-Free Extra Strength Tablets *(acetaminophen)*	OK	L1			
Anacin Max Strength Tablets / Regular Strength Tablets *(aspirin / caffeine)*	UNSAFE	L4			
Arnicare Leg Cramps *(Arnica montana / homeopathic herbs)*	OK	L3			
Arthritis pain relief caplets, generic *(acetaminophen)*	OK	L1			
Ascriptin Maximum Strength Tablets / Regular Strength Tablets *(aluminum-magnesium hydroxide / aspirin / calcium carbonate)*	UNSAFE	L4			

	SAFETY LEVEL (P. 19)		MONITOR INFANT FOR DROWSINESS OR EXCITABILITY	LOOK FOR ALTERNATIVE THAT DOES NOT COMBINE INGREDIENTS	MONITOR MILK SUPPLY & DRINK EXTRA FLUIDS
Aspirin 325 mg tablets, generic *(aspirin)*	UNSAFE	L4			
Aspirin 500 mg tablets, generic *(aspirin)*	UNSAFE	L4			
Aspirin-free pain relief tablets, generic *(acetaminophen)*	OK	L1			
AZO Urinary Pain Relief Maximum Strength Tablets / Urinary Pain Relief Tablets *(phenazopyridine)*	OK	L3			
AZO Urinary Tract Defense *(methenamine / sodium salicylate)*	UNSAFE	L4			
Back Quell Tablets *(acetaminophen / magnesium salicylate)*	UNSAFE	L4			
Bayer Back & Body Pain Caplets / Headache Caplets *(aspirin / caffeine)*	UNSAFE	L4			
Bayer Extra Strength Caplets / Genuine Aspirin Tablets / Safety Coated Caplets *(aspirin)*	UNSAFE	L4			
BC Arthritis Powders / Original Powders *(aspirin / caffeine)*	UNSAFE	L4			
Bromo-Seltzer Powders *(acetaminophen / citric acid / sodium bicarbonate)*	OK	L1		*	
Bufferin Tablets *(aspirin / calcium-magnesium carbonate / magnesium oxide)*	UNSAFE	L4			
Cramp 911 Roll-on Lotion *(homeopathic herbs)*	OK	L3			
Cystex UTI Pain Relief Tablets *(methenamine / sodium salicylate)*	UNSAFE	L4			
Datril Tablets *(acetaminophen)*	OK	L1			
Doan's Extra Strength Caplets *(magnesium salicylate)*	UNSAFE	L4			
Ecotrin Regular Strength Tablets *(aspirin)*	UNSAFE	L4			
Emagrin Tablets *(aspirin / caffeine / salicylamide)*	UNSAFE	L4			
Empirin Tablets *(aspirin)*	UNSAFE	L4			

		SAFETY LEVEL (P. 19)	MONITOR INFANT FOR DROWSINESS OR EXCITABILITY	LOOK FOR ALTERNATIVE THAT DOES NOT COMBINE INGREDIENTS	MONITOR MILK SUPPLY & DRINK EXTRA FLUIDS
Excedrin Back & Body Capsules *(acetaminophen / aspirin buffered)*	UNSAFE	L4			
Excedrin Extra Strength Caplets / Extra Strength Express Gels / Extra Strength Geltabs / Extra Strength Tablets *(acetaminophen / aspirin)*	UNSAFE	L4			
Excedrin Migraine Caplets / Migraine Geltabs / Migraine Tablets *(acetaminophen / aspirin)*	UNSAFE	L4			
Excedrin Tension Headache Caplets / Tension Headache Express Gels / Tension Headache Geltabs *(acetaminophen / caffeine)*	OK	L2	*	*	
Goody's Back & Body Pain Powder *(acetaminophen / aspirin)*	UNSAFE	L4			
Goody's Cool Orange Powder / Extra Strength Headache Powder / Mixed Fruit Blast Powder *(acetaminophen / aspirin / caffeine)*	UNSAFE	L4			
Haltran Tablets *(ibuprofen)*	OK	L1			
Hyland's Leg Cramps Tablets *(homeopathic herbs / magnesium / quinine)*	UNSAFE	L4			
Hyland's Restful Legs Tablets *(homeopathic herbs / sulfur / zinc)*	UNSAFE	L4			
Ibuprofen 200 mg tablets, generic *(ibuprofen)*	OK	L1			
Ibuprohm Max Tablets / Tablets *(ibuprofen)*	OK	L1			
MagniLife Relaxing Legs Tablets *(homeopathic herbs)*	OK	L3			
Magsal Tablets *(magnesium salicylate / phenyltoloxamine)*	UNSAFE	L4			
Midol Complete Caffeine Free Caplets *(acetaminophen / pamabrom / pyrilamine)*	UNSAFE	L4			
Midol Complete Caplets / Complete Gelcaps *(acetaminophen / caffeine / pyrilamine)*	OK	L3	*	*	

		SAFETY LEVEL (P. 19)	MONITOR INFANT FOR DROWSINESS OR EXCITABILITY	LOOK FOR ALTERNATIVE THAT DOES NOT COMBINE INGREDIENTS	MONITOR MILK SUPPLY & DRINK EXTRA FLUIDS
Mobigesic Tablets *(magnesium salicylate / phenyltoloxamine)*	UNSAFE	L4			
Motrin IB Caplets / Tablets *(ibuprofen)*	OK	L1			
Pamprin Max Pain + Energy Caplets *(acetaminophen / aspirin / caffeine)*	UNSAFE	L4			
Pamprin Multi-Symptom Caplets *(acetaminophen / pamabrom / pyrilamine)*	UNSAFE	L4			
Panadol Extra Tablets *(acetaminophen / caffeine)*	OK	L2	*	*	
Panadol Tablets *(acetaminophen)*	OK	L1			
Percogesic Extra Strength Caplets / Original Strength Caplets *(acetaminophen / phenyltoloxamine)*	UNSAFE	L4			
Premsyn PMS Caplets *(acetaminophen / pamabrom / pyrilamine)*	UNSAFE	L4			
Prodium Tablets *(phenazopyridine)*	OK	L3			
Re-Azo Tablets *(phenazopyridine)*	OK	L3			
Stanback Headache Powders *(aspirin / caffeine / salicylamide)*	UNSAFE	L4			
Supac Tablets *(acetaminophen / aspirin / caffeine)*	UNSAFE	L4			
Traumeel Oral Drops *(Arnica montana / homeopathic herbs)*	UNSAFE	L4			
Traumeel Oral Liquid in vials *(Arnica montana / homeopathic herbs)*	UNSAFE	L4			
Traumeel Tablets *(Arnica montana / homeopathic herbs)*	UNSAFE	L4			
Tylenol 8 Hour Arthritis Pain Caplets / 8 Hour Caplets *(acetaminophen)*	OK	L1			
Tylenol Extra Strength Caplets / Extra Strength Coated Tablets / Extra Strength Cool Caplets / Extra Strength Rapid-Release Gelcaps *(acetaminophen)*	OK	L1			

		SAFETY LEVEL (P. 19)	MONITOR INFANT FOR DROWSINESS OR EXCITABILITY	LOOK FOR ALTERNATIVE THAT DOES NOT COMBINE INGREDIENTS	MONITOR MILK SUPPLY & DRINK EXTRA FLUIDS
Tylenol For Children + Adults Oral Suspension / Regular Strength Liquid Gels / Regular Strength Tablets *(acetaminophen)*	OK	L1			
Uricalm Intensive *(acetaminophen / aspirin / caffeine)*	UNSAFE	L4			
Uricalm Max *(phenazopyridine)*	OK	L1			
Uristat Tablets *(phenazopyridine)*	OK	L3			
Vanquish Caplets *(acetaminophen / aspirin / caffeine)*	UNSAFE	L4			

Antacid, Antiflatulent, Digestive Aid, and Heartburn Relief Products

		SAFETY LEVEL (PAGE 19)
Alka-Seltzer Extra Strength Tablets / Lemon Lime Tablets / Original Tablets *(aspirin / citric acid / sodium bicarbonate)*	UNSAFE	L4
Alka-Seltzer Gold Tablets *(citric acid / potassium bicarbonate / sodium bicarbonate)*	OK	L1
Alka-Seltzer Heartburn Relief Tablets *(citric acid / sodium bicarbonate)*	OK	L1
AlternaGEL Liquid *(aluminum hydroxide)*	OK	L1
Aluminum carbonate liquid, generic *(aluminum carbonate)*	OK	L1
Aluminum hydroxide gel, generic *(aluminum hydroxide)*	OK	L1
BD Lactinex Dietary Supplement Granules / Tablets *(lactobacillus culture)*	OK	L1
Beano Food Enzyme Dietary Supplemental Drops / Tablets *(alpha-galactosidase enzyme)*	OK	L1
Beano Meltaways / Tablets *(enzymes / sorbitol)*	OK	L1
Brioschi Powders *(sodium bicarbonate / tartaric acid)*	OK	L1
CharcoCaps Anti-Gas Formula Capsules *(activated charcoal)*	OK	L1
Chooz Gum *(calcium carbonate)*	OK	L1
Citrocarbonate Effervescent Antacid Salts *(sodium bicarbonate-citrate)*	OK	L1
DDS-1 acidophilus capsules, generic *(lactobacillus acidophilus)*	OK	L1
Di-Gel Tablets *(calcium carbonate / magnesium hydroxide / simethicone)*	OK	L1
EZ-Char Activated Charcoal Pellets *(activated charcoal)*	OK	L1
GasAid Maximum Strength Anti-Gas Softgels *(simethicone)*	OK	L1
Gas-X Antigas Chewable Tablets / Antigas Softgels / Antigas Thin Strips *(simethicone)*	OK	L1
Gas-X Extra Strength with Maalox Chewable Tablets *(calcium carbonate / simethicone)*	OK	L1
Gaviscon Extra Strength Liquid / Extra Strength Tablets / Regular Strength Liquid / Regular Strength Tablets *(aluminum hydroxide / magnesium carbonate)*	OK	L1

		SAFETY LEVEL (PAGE 19)
Gelusil Antacid & Anti-gas Chewable Tablets *(aluminum-magnesium hydroxide / simethicone)*	OK	L1
Lactaid Fast Act Capsules / Fast Act Chewable Tablets / Original Tablets *(lactase)*	OK	L1
Lactase enzyme capsules / liquid drops, generic *(lactase)*	OK	L1
Maalox Advanced Maximum Strength Chewable Tablets *(calcium carbonate / simethicone)*	OK	L1
Maalox Advanced Maximum Strength Liquid / Advanced Regular Strength Liquid *(aluminum-magnesium hydroxide / simethicone)*	OK	L1
Maalox Regular Strength Chewable Tablets *(calcium carbonate)*	OK	L1
Maalox Total Relief Maximum Strength Relief Liquid *(bismuth subsalicylate)*	UNSAFE	L4
Mylanta Coat & Cool Liquid / Tonight Liquid *(calcium carbonate / magnesium hydroxide / simethicone)*	OK	L1
Mylanta Gas Minis Chewable Tablets *(simethicone)*	OK	L1
Mylanta Maximum Strength Liquid *(aluminum-magnesium hydroxide / simethicone)*	OK	L1
Mylanta ONE Tablets *(calcium carbonate / magnesium hydroxide / simethicone)*	OK	L1
Nature's Way Lactase Enzyme *(lactase)*	OK	L1
Nexium 24 HR *(esomeprazole)*	OK	L2
Nizatidine tablets, generic *(nizatidine)*	OK	L2
Pepcid AC Maximum Strength Tablets / Original Strength Tablets *(famotidine)*	OK	L2
Pepcid Complete Chewable Tablets *(calcium carbonate / famotidine / magnesium carbonate)*	OK	L2
Pepto Bismol Cherry Chewable Tablets / Cherry Liquid / LiquiCaps / Original Caplets / Original Chewable Tablets / Original Liquid *(bismuth subsalicylate)*	UNSAFE	L4
Pepto Bismol Cherry Ultra Liquid / Ultra Caplets / Ultra Liquid / Ultra with InstaCOOL Liquid *(bismuth subsalicylate)*	UNSAFE	L4
Phazyme Ultra Strength Anti-Gas Fast Gels *(simethicone)*	OK	L1
Phillips' Milk of Magnesia Suspension *(magnesium hydroxide)*	OK	L1
Prevacid 24 HR *(lansoprazole)*	OK	L2

		SAFETY LEVEL (PAGE 19)
Prilosec OTC Tablets *(omeprazole)*	OK	L2
Riopan Plus Suspension / Plus Tablets *(magaldrate / simethicone)*	OK	L1
Rolaids Advanced Plus Anti-Gas Chewable Tablets / Softchews *(calcium carbonate / magnesium hydroxide / simethicone)*	OK	L1
Rolaids Antacid & Antigas Soft Chews *(calcium carbonate / simethicone)*	OK	L1
Rolaids Extra Strength Chewable Tablets / Ultra Strength Chewable Tablets / Ultra Strength Softchews *(calcium carbonate / magnesium hydroxide)*	OK	L1
Schiff's Digestive Advantage Daily Probiotic Capsules *(Bacillus coagulans)*	OK	L3
Sodium bicarbonate powder / tablets, generic *(sodium bicarbonate)*	OK	L1
Tagamet HB 200 Tablets *(cimetidine)*	OK	L2
TUMS Chewable Tablets / Smoothies Chewable Tablets *(calcium carbonate)*	OK	L1
TUMS Extra Strength 750 Chewable Tablets / Extra Strength 750 Chewy Bites / Extra Strength 750 Sugar-Free Chewable Tablets *(calcium carbonate)*	OK	L1
TUMS Ultra Strength 1000 Chewable Tablets *(calcium carbonate)*	OK	L1
Zantac 75 Tablets / 150 Tablets *(ranitidine)*	OK	L2
Zegerid OTC Tablets *(omeprazole / sodium bicarbonate)*	OK	L2

Antidiarrheal Preparations

		SAFETY LEVEL (PAGE 19)	DO NOT USE MORE THAN TWO DAYS IN A ROW
Equalactin Chewable Tablets *(calcium polycarbophil)*	OK	L1	
FiberCon Caplets *(calcium polycarbophil)*	OK	L1	
Hyland's Diarrex Tablets *(homeopathic herbs)*	UNSAFE	L4	
Imodium A-D Caplets / E-Z Chews / Liquid *(loperamide)*	OK	L2	*
Imodium Multi-Symptom Relief Caplets / Multi-Symptom Relief Chewable Tablets *(loperamide / simethicone)*	OK	L2	*
Kaopectate Caplets / Liquid / MAX Liquid *(bismuth subsalicylate)*	UNSAFE	L4	
Konsyl Psyllium Fiber Caplets *(psyllium)*	OK	L1	
Maalox Total Relief Liquid *(bismuth subsalicylate)*	UNSAFE	L3	
Pepto Bismol Caplets / Chewable Tablets / Liquid / Liquid Max *(bismuth subsalicylate)*	UNSAFE	L4	
Pepto Diarrhea Caplets / LiquiCaps / Liquid *(bismuth subsalicylate)*	UNSAFE	L4	
Rheaban Maximum Strength Tablets *(attapulgite)*	OK	L1	

Asthma Preparations

For all OTC asthma products, *it is highly recommended to consult with a health-care provider prior to use*. Products below are not marked as OK or UNSAFE because definitive safety information cannot be provided here.

Information Capsule:

 If using prescription **THEOPHYLLINE**-containing asthma products, mothers should avoid consuming chocolate, tea, coffee, or caffeinated soda in order to prevent excessive stimulation of the infant (e.g., restlessness, insomnia).

	SAFETY LEVEL (PAGE 19)
Asthmahaler Mist Inhaler *(epinephrine)*	L1
Asthmanephrin Mist Inhaler *(epinephrine)*	L1
Bronkaid Caplets *(ephedrine / guaifenesin)*	L4
Bronkaid Mist Inhaler *(epinephrine)*	L1
Bronkotabs *(ephedrine / guaifenesin)*	L4
Primatene Mist Inhaler *(epinephrine)*	L1
Primatene Tablets *(ephedrine / guaifenesin)*	L4
Respitrol Liquid *(herbs)*	L4

Callus, Corn, and Wart Products

		SAFETY LEVEL (PAGE 19)	AVOID BREATHING FUMES
Compound W Fast-Acting Gel / Fast-Acting Liquid *(salicylic acid)*	OK	L2	*
Compound W Freeze Off *(dimethyl ether / propane)*	OK	L2	*
Compound W NitroFreeze *(nitrous oxide)*	OK	L3	*
Compound W One Step Invisible Strips / One Step Pads *(salicylic acid)*	OK	L2	*
Corn removal plasters, generic *(salicylic acid)*	OK	L2	*
Curad Mediplast Pads *(salicylic acid)*	OK	L2	*
Dr. Scholl's Callus Removers / Corn and Callus Removers / Corn Removers *(salicylic acid)*	OK	L2	*
Dr. Scholl's Clear Away Wart Removers *(salicylic acid)*	OK	L2	*
Dr. Scholl's Freeze Away Max Wart Remover / Freeze Away Wart Remover *(dimethyl ether / propane)*	OK	L2	*
Durasal Wart Remover Solution *(salicylic acid)*	OK	L2	*
Duofilm Salicylic Acid Wart Remover Liquid *(salicylic acid)*	OK	L2	*
Freezone Liquid Corn and Callus Remover *(salicylic acid)*	OK	L2	*
Gordofilm Wart Remover Solution *(salicylic acid)*	OK	L2	*
Hydrisalic gel, generic *(salicylic acid)*	OK	L2	*
Keralyt Gel *(salicylic acid)*	OK	L2	*
Liquid wart remover, generic *(salicylic acid)*	OK	L2	*
Mosco Callus & Corn Remover Liquid *(salicylic acid)*	OK	L2	*
Occlusal-HP Topical Wart Remover *(salicylic acid)*	OK	L2	*
PEDiNOL Sal-Plant Gel *(salicylic acid)*	OK	L2	*
ProVent Wart Remover *(homeopathic herbs)*	OK	L2	*
Salicylic acid film / gel / liquid, generic *(salicylic acid)*	OK	L2	*
Tinamed Wart Remover *(salicylic acid)*	OK	L2	*
Wartner Freezing Wart Remover *(dimethyl ether / propane)*	OK	L2	*
WartStick *(salicylic acid)*	OK	L2	*

* *Additional note applies*

OK *OK to use*   UNSAFE *Do not use*

Cold and Cough Inhalers, Lozenges, Rubs, and Sprays

		SAFETY LEVEL (PAGE 19)	MONITOR INFANT FOR DROWSINESS
Benzedrex Inhaler (propylhexedrine)	UNSAFE	L5	
Burt's Bees Lozenges (eucalyptus / honey / menthol)	OK	L2	
Cepacol Sore Throat Lozenges / Sore Throat Spray (benzocaine / menthol)	OK	L2	
Cepastat Sore Throat Lozenges (eucalyptus / menthol / phenol)	UNSAFE	L4	
Chloraseptic Sore Throat Lozenges (benzocaine / menthol)	OK	L2	
Chloraseptic Sore Throat Spray (phenol)	UNSAFE	L4	
Cold-EEZE Lozenges (zinc)	OK	L1	
Cold-EEZE Plus Defense Lozenges (homeopathic herbs / zinc)	OK	L3	
Fisherman's Friend Menthol Cough Suppressant Lozenges (menthol)	OK	L1	
HALLS Breezers (pectin)	OK	L1	
HALLS Defense Cough Drops (vitamin C)	OK	L1	
HALLS Relief Cough Drops (eucalyptus / menthol)	OK	L2	
HALLS Soothe Cough Drops (honey / menthol)	OK	L2	
Luden's Cough Drops (menthol / pectin)	OK	L1	
Maty's All Natural Vapor Rub (apple cider vinegar / clove oil / coriander / ginger / honey / turmeric)	OK	L1	
Mentholatum Nighttime Vaporizing Rub (camphor / eucalyptus / menthol)	OK	L2	
Mentholatum Ointment (methyl salicylate)	OK	L3	
Mentholatum Original Ointment (camphor / menthol)	OK	L2	
Nature's Way Sambucus Organic Zinc Lozenges (elderberry / zinc)	OK	L1	
N'ICE Lozenges (menthol)	OK	L1	
Pine Brothers Softish Throat Drops (glycerin / honey)	OK	L1	

		SAFETY LEVEL (PAGE 19)	MONITOR INFANT FOR DROWSINESS
Ricola Original Herb Cough Drops *(menthol / multiple herbs)*	OK	L1	
Sambucol Black Elderberry Lozenges *(elderberry / honey / vitamin C / zinc)*	OK	L1	
Sucrets Sore Throat & Cough Lozenges *(dyclonine / menthol / vitamin C / zinc)*	OK	L3	
Sucrets Sore Throat, Cough & Dry Mouth Lozenge *(dyclonine / menthol / pectin / vitamin C / zinc)*	OK	L3	
Sucrets Sore Throat Lozenges *(dyclonine)*	OK	L3	
TheraZinc Lozenges *(elderberry / zinc)*	OK	L1	
Vicks VapoBath / VapoShower / VapoSteam *(camphor / eucalyptus / menthol)*	OK	L2	
Vicks VapoCool Sore Throat Relief Lozenges / VapoCool Sore Throat Spray *(benzocaine / menthol)*	OK	L2	
Vicks VapoCream / VapoPatch / VapoRub *(camphor / eucalyptus / menthol)*	OK	L2	
Vicks VapoDrops Cough Relief Drops *(menthol)*	OK	L1	
Vicks VapoInhaler *(camphor / menthol / methyl salicylate / siberian fir)*	OK	L3	*
Zarbee's 96% Honey Cough Soothers + Immune Support *(elderberry / honey / vitamin C / vitamin D / zinc)*	OK	L1	
Zarbee's 96% Honey Cough Soothers + Mucus *(honey / ivy leaf / menthol)*	OK	L3	
Zarbee's 99% Honey Cough Soothers *(honey)*	OK	L1	
Zicam Cold Remedy Lozenges *(zinc)*	OK	L1	

Dandruff, Psoriasis, and Seborrhea Scalp Treatment Products

		SAFETY LEVEL (PAGE 19)
Dandrex Shampoo (selenium sulfide)	OK	L3
Denorex Dandruff Daily Protection Shampoo (pyrithione zinc)	OK	L2
Denorex Dandruff Extra Strength Shampoo (salicylic acid)	OK	L2
Denorex Therapeutic Protection 2-in-1 Shampoo / Therapeutic Protection Shampoo (coal tar)	OK	L3
Dermarest Psoriasis Medicated Moisturizer / Psoriasis Medicated Overnight Treatment / Psoriasis Medicated Shampoo-Conditioner / Psoriasis Medicated Skin Treatment / Psoriasis Scalp Treatment (salicylic acid)	OK	L2
DHS Sal Shampoo (salicylic acid)	OK	L2
DHS Tar Gel Shampoo / Tar Shampoo (coal tar)	OK	L3
DHS Zinc Shampoo (pyrithione zinc)	OK	L2
Head & Shoulders Aloe Vera 2-in-1 Dandruff Shampoo + Conditioner / Aloe Vera Dandruff Shampoo (aloe / pyrithione zinc)	OK	L3
Head & Shoulders Apple Cider Vinegar 2-in-1 Dandruff Shampoo + Conditioner / Apple Cider Vinegar Dandruff Shampoo (apple cider vinegar / pyrithione zinc)	OK	L2
Head & Shoulders Classic Clean 2-in-1 Dandruff Shampoo + Conditioner / Classic Clean Dandruff Conditioner / Classic Clean Dandruff Shampoo (pyrithione zinc)	OK	L2
Head & Shoulders Clinical Strength Dandruff Defense + Advanced Oil Control Shampoo (selenium sulfide)	OK	L2
Head & Shoulders Clinical Strength Dandruff Defense Intensive Itch Relief Shampoo (menthol / peppermint oil / selenium sulfide)	OK	L2
Head & Shoulders Clinical Strength Dandruff Defense Sensitive Scalp Shampoo (aloe / selenium sulfide)	OK	L3
Head & Shoulders Dry Scalp Care 2-in-1 Dandruff Shampoo + Conditioner / Dry Scalp Care Dandruff Conditioner / Dry Scalp Care Dandruff Shampoo (pyrithione zinc / sweet almond oil)	OK	L2
Head & Shoulders Itchy Scalp Care Dandruff Shampoo (eucalyptus / menthol / peppermint oil)	OK	L2

		SAFETY LEVEL (PAGE 19)
Head & Shoulders Lemon Oil Anti-Dandruff 2-in-1 Shampoo + Conditioner *(lemon / menthol / pyrithione zinc)*	OK	L2
Head & Shoulders Supreme Color Protect Conditioner / Supreme Color Protect Shampoo *(pyrithione zinc)*	OK	L2
Head & Shoulders Volume Boost Dandruff Conditioner / Volume Boost Dandruff Shampoo *(menthol / pyrithione zinc)*	OK	L2
Ionil Plus Conditioning Shampoo *(salicylic acid)*	OK	L2
Ionil-T Plus Shampoo / Shampoo *(coal tar)*	OK	L3
La Roche-Posay Kerium DS Anti-Dandruff Cream Shampoo for Dry Scalp / Kerium DS Anti-Dandruff Gel Shampoo for Oily Scalp *(coco betaine / capryloyl salicylic acid / salicylic acid)*	OK	L2
MG217 Psoriasis Gel / Ointment / Shampoo *(coal tar)*	OK	L3
MG217 Psoriasis Shampoo + Conditioner *(salicylic acid)*	OK	L2
Neutrogena T/Gel Therapeutic Shampoo Extra Strength / T/Gel Therapeutic Shampoo Original Formula *(coal tar)*	OK	L3
Neutrogena T/Sal Therapeutic Shampoo Scalp Build-Up Control *(salicylic acid)*	OK	L2
Nizoral Anti-Dandruff Shampoo *(ketoconazole)*	OK	L2
P&S Liquid / Shampoo *(glycerin / mineral oil)*	OK	L1
Pantene Pro-V Anti-Dandruff Shampoo *(pyrithione zinc)*	OK	L2
Pert Plus Classic Clean Anti-Dandruff 2-in-1 Shampoo + Conditioner *(pyrithione zinc)*	OK	L2
Psoriasin Daytime Relief Vanishing Gel / Deep Moisturizing Ointment *(coal tar)*	OK	L3
Scalpicin Maximum Strength Scalp Itch Relief Liquid *(hydrocortisone)*	OK	L2
Sebex Medicated Dandruff, Seborrheic Dermatitis & Psoriasis Shampoo *(salicylic acid / sulfur)*	OK	L2
Sebulex Medicated Dandruff Shampoo *(salicylic acid / sulfur)*	OK	L2
Selsun blue Daily Care Itchy Dry Scalp Antidandruff Shampoo *(aloe / pyrithione zinc)*	OK	L2
Selsun blue Maximum Strength 2-in-1 Antidandruff Shampoo & Conditioner / Maximum Strength Medicated Antidandruff Shampoo *(selenium sulfide)*	OK	L3

		SAFETY LEVEL (PAGE 19)
Selsun blue Maximum Strength Moisturizing Antidandruff Shampoo (aloe / selenium sulfide)	OK	L3
Selsun blue Naturals Daily Care Itchy Dry Scalp Antidandruff Shampoo (acacia / aloe / chamomile / lavender / rosemary / salicylic acid)	OK	L2
Suave Essentials Scalp Control Anti-Dandruff 2-in-1 Shampoo + Conditioner / Essentials Scalp Control Deep Clean Anti-Dandruff Shampoo (pyrithione zinc)	OK	L2
Zincon Medicated Dandruff Shampoo (pyrithione zinc)	OK	L2

Heart Attack and Stroke Risk Reduction Agents

		SAFETY LEVEL (PAGE 19)
Bayer Chewable Low Dose Aspirin Regimen Tablets / Low Dose Safety Coated Aspirin Regimen Tablets *(81 mg aspirin)*	OK	L3
Ecotrin 81 mg Low Strength Safety Coated Aspirin Tablets *(81 mg aspirin)*	OK	L3
Halfprin 81 mg Tablets *(81 mg aspirin)*	OK	L3
Low-dose aspirin tablets, generic *(81 mg aspirin)*	OK	L3
St. Joseph Low Dose Aspirin Chewable Tablets / Low Dose Aspirin Safety (Enteric) Coated Tablets *(81 mg aspirin)*	OK	L3

Hemorrhoidal Preparations

Information Capsules:

 Topical hemorrhoidal preparations are used for their local effect, therefore, their use should not result in large amounts of the active ingredient getting into breastmilk.

 Topical preparations include **HYDROCORTISONE**, **COCOA BUTTER**, **WITCH HAZEL**, various oils, **GLYCERIN**, and other ingredients.

		SAFETY LEVEL (PAGE 19)
Americaine Hemorrhoidal Ointment *(benzocaine)*	OK	L2
Anusol-HC Ointment / Suppositories *(hydrocortisone)*	OK	L2
Balneol Hygienic Cleansing Lotion *(lanolin oil / mineral oil / moisturizers)*	OK	L1
Calmol 4 Hemorrhoidal Suppositories *(cocoa butter / zinc oxide)*	OK	L1
Citrucel with Methylcellulose Fiber Caplets / Fiber Powder *(methylcellulose)*	OK	L1
Colace Clear Stool Softener Soft Gels / Regular Strength Stool Softener Capsules *(docusate sodium)*	OK	L2
Dibucaine ointment, generic *(dibucaine)*	OK	L3
Docusol Constipation Relief Mini Enemas *(docusate sodium)*	OK	L2
Dulcolax Stimulant-Free Stool Softener Liquid Gels *(docusate sodium)*	OK	L2
Enemeez Regular Mini Enema *(docusate sodium)*	OK	L2
Equalactin Laxative Chewable Tablets *(calcium polycarbophil)*	OK	L1
FiberCon Caplets *(calcium polycarbophil)*	OK	L1
Hyland's Hemorrhoids *(homeopathic herbs)*	OK	L3
Kaopectate Liqui-Gels *(docusate calcium)*	OK	L2
Konsyl Daily Fiber Gummies *(chicory root fiber)*	OK	L1
Konsyl Daily Psyllium Fiber Capsules / Daily Psyllium Fiber Orange Sugar Free Supplement Powder / Daily Psyllium Fiber Supplement Powder *(psyllium)*	OK	L1

		SAFETY LEVEL (PAGE 19)
Metamucil 3-in-1 Fiber Capsules / 4-in-1 Fiber Sugar-Free Smooth Powder / 4-in-1 Fiber Real Sugar Smooth Powder / 4-in-1 Fiber Real Sugar Coarse Powder / Fiber Thins / Premium Blend Sugar-Free Fiber Powder *(psyllium)*	OK	L1
Peterson's Ointment *(methysalicylate)*	OK	L3
Phillips' Stool Softener Liquid Gels *(docusate sodium)*	OK	L2
Pramoxine HCl 1% hemorrhoidal foam, generic *(pramoxine)*	OK	L1
Preparation H Hemorrhoidal Cooling Gel *(phenylephrine / witch hazel)*	OK	L3
Preparation H Hemorrhoidal Cream Multi-Symptom Maximum Strength Pain Relief *(glycerin / phenylephrine / pramoxine / white petrolatum)*	OK	L3
Preparation H Hemorrhoidal Ointment *(mineral oil / petrolatum / phenylephrine / shark liver oil)*	OK	L3
Preparation H Hemorrhoidal Suppositories *(cocoa butter / phenylephrine / shark liver oil)*	OK	L3
Preparation H Medicated Wipes *(witch hazel)*	OK	L1
Preparation H Soothing Relief Anti-Itch Cream *(hydrocortisone)*	OK	L2
RectiCare Advanced Hemorrhoidal Cream *(lidocaine / mineral oil / phenylephrine / white petrolatum)*	OK	L2
RectiCare Anorectal Cream *(lidocaine)*	OK	L2
T.N. Dickinson's Witch Hazel Hemorrhoidal Pads *(witch hazel)*	OK	L1
Tronolane Anesthetic Hemorrhoidal Cream *(pramoxine / zinc oxide)*	OK	L1
Tucks Medicated Cooling Pads *(glycerin / witch hazel)*	OK	L1

✳ *Additional note applies*   119   OK *OK to use*   UNSAFE *Do not use*

Insulin Preparations

Information Capsules:

 The use of **INSULIN** is common in pregnant women, both for those previously diagnosed with diabetes and those who develop gestational diabetes during pregnancy. After the birth of the infant, the need for insulin may or may not still remain. As a result, breastfeeding dose modifications are usually necessary.

 Under the guidance of a physician, the dose of insulin should be reduced by approximately 25% of the prepregnancy dose in order to prevent hypoglycemic reactions in the breastfeeding parent. It is recommended to moderately increase carbohydrate intake as well.

 While breastfeeding, there should be no effects of insulin on the infant. Insulin is degraded in the gastrointestinal tract and does not readily pass into breastmilk.

Note that nonprescription insulin preparations may not be available everywhere, and are not equivalent to prescription preparations. It is extremely important to talk to a healthcare provider before using nonprescription insulin.

	SAFETY LEVEL (PAGE 19)		SPECIAL NOTES
All insulin preparations	OK	L1	Consult a physician before using OTC preparations. During breastfeeding it is recommended that the insulin dose be reduced by 25% of the prepregnancy dose.
Glutose 15 / Glutose 45 (oral glucose gel for treatment of insulin reaction)	OK	L1	

OK *OK to use*   UNSAFE *Do not use*   120   * *Additional note applies*

Laxatives and Stool Softeners

		SAFETY LEVEL (PAGE 19)	DO NOT USE FOR MORE THAN 1 OR 2 DOSES
Alophen Enteric Coated Stimulant Laxative Pills (bisacodyl)	OK	L2	*
Benefiber Original Prebiotic Fiber Supplement (wheat dextrin)	OK	L1	
Bisacodyl tablets, generic (bisacodyl)	OK	L2	*
Cascara sagrada tablets, generic (cascara sagrada)	UNSAFE	L3	
Castor oil, generic (castor oil)	UNSAFE	L3	
Ceo-Two Laxative Suppositories (potassium bitartrate / sodium bicarbonate)	OK	L2	*
Charak Pharma Regulax Forte Tablets (herbs)	UNSAFE	L4	
Citrucel with Methylcellulose Fiber Caplets / Fiber Powder (methylcellulose)	OK	L1	
Colace 2-in-1 Stool Softener + Stimulant Laxative Tablets (docusate / sennosides)	OK	L3	*
Colace Clear Stool Softener Soft Gels / Regular Strength Stool Softener Capsules (docusate sodium)	OK	L2	
Colace Glycerin Suppositories (glycerin)	OK	L2	*
Correctol Tablets (bisacodyl)	OK	L2	*
Docusate calcium stool softener, generic (docusate calcium)	OK	L2	
Docusol Constipation Relief Mini Enemas (docusate sodium)	OK	L2	
Doxidan Tablets (bisacodyl)	OK	L2	*
DulcoEase Capsules (docusate sodium)	OK	L2	
Dulcolax Chewy Fruit Bites / Liquid Laxative / Soft Chews (magnesium hydroxide)	OK	L1	
Dulcolax Medicated Laxative Suppositories / Overnight Relief Laxative Tablets (bisacodyl)	OK	L2	*
Dulcolax Stimulant-Free Stool Softener Liquid Gels (docusate sodium)	OK	L2	
Epsom salt saline laxative, generic (magnesium sulfate)	OK	L1	*
Equalactin Chewable Tablets (calcium polycarbophil)	OK	L1	

		SAFETY LEVEL (PAGE 19)	DO NOT USE FOR MORE THAN 1 OR 2 DOSES
Ex-Lax Maximum Strength Tablets / Regular Strength Tablets (sennosides)	OK	L3	*
Fiberall Powder (psyllium)	OK	L1	
Fibercon Caplets (calcium polycarbophil)	OK	L1	
Fleet Bisacodyl Enema (bisacodyl)	OK	L2	*
Fleet Enema Extra / Saline Enema (dibasic sodium phosphate / monobasic sodium phosphate)	OK	L1	*
Fleet Glycerin Suppositories (glycerin)	OK	L1	
Fleet Mineral Oil Enema (mineral oil)	OK	L1	*
Hydrocil Instant Fiber Laxative Powder (psyllium)	OK	L1	
Innerclean Herbal Blend Tablets (herbs / psyllium / senna)	OK	L3	*
Kaopectate Liqui-Gels (docusate calcium)	OK	L1	
Kondremul Lubricant Laxative Emulsion (mineral oil)	OK	L1	*
Konsyl Daily Fiber Gummies (chicory root fiber)	OK	L1	
Konsyl Daily Psyllium Fiber Capsules / Daily Psyllium Fiber Orange Sugar Free Supplement Powder / Daily Psyllium Fiber Supplement Powder (psyllium)	OK	L1	
Magnesium citrate solution, generic (magnesium citrate)	OK	L1	*
Malt soup extract, generic (malt soup extract powder / potassium sorbate / sodium propionate)	OK	L1	
Metamucil 3-in-1 Fiber Capsules / 4-in-1 Fiber Real Sugar Coarse Powder / 4-in-1 Fiber Real Sugar Smooth Powder / 4-in-1 Fiber Sugar-Free Smooth Powder / Fiber Thins / Premium Blend Sugar-Free Fiber Powder (psyllium)	OK	L1	
MiraLAX Powder (PEG-3350)	OK	L3	*
Perdiem Overnight Relief Tablets (sennosides)	OK	L3	*
Phillips' Laxative Caplets (magnesium)	OK	L1	*
Phillips' Milk of Magnesia Liquid (magnesium hydroxide)	OK	L1	
Phillips' Stool Softener Liquid Gels (docusate sodium)	OK	L1	
Senokot Dietary Supplement Laxative Gummies (senna)	OK	L3	*
Senokot Extra Strength Tablets / Regular Strength Tablets (sennosides)	OK	L3	*

		SAFETY LEVEL (PAGE 19)	DO NOT USE FOR MORE THAN 1 OR 2 DOSES
Senokot Laxative Tea *(chamomile / senna)*	OK	L3	✱
Senokot-S Dual Action Tablets *(docusate / sennosides)*	OK	L3	✱
Shaklee Herb-Lax Tablets *(herbs / senna)*	OK	L3	✱

Motion Sickness, Nausea, and Vomiting Relief Products

		SAFETY LEVEL (PAGE 19)	MONITOR INFANT FOR DROWSINESS
Benadryl Allergy Dye-Free Antihistamine Liqui-Gels / Allergy Extra Strength Ultratabs Antihistamine Tablets / Allergy Ultratabs Antihistamine Tablets *(diphenhydramine)*	OK	L2	*
Bonine for Motion Sickness Chewable Tablets *(meclizine)*	OK	L3	*
Dramamine Motion Sickness All Day Less Drowsy Tablets / Motion Sickness Less Drowsy Chewable Tablets / Nausea Long Lasting Tablets *(meclizine)*	OK	L3	*
Dramamine Motion Sickness Chewable Tablets / Motion Sickness Original Tablets *(dimenhydrinate)*	OK	L2	*
Dramamine Motion Sickness Non-Drowsy Natural Ginger / Nausea Ginger Chews / Nausea Multipurpose Tablets *(ginger)*	OK	L1	
Emetrol Non-Drowsy Rapid Nausea Relief Chewables *(diphenhydramine)*	OK	L2	*
Emetrol Non-Drowsy Rapid Nausea Relief Syrup *(dextrose / levulose / phosphoric acid)*	OK	L1	
Humco Cola Syrup *(cola syrup)*	OK	L1	
Motion sickness relief tablets with dimenhydrinate, generic *(dimenhydrinate)*	OK	L2	*
MotionEaze All-Natural Motion Sickness Relief Topical Oil *(herbs)*	UNSAFE	L4	
Nauzene Chewable Tablets *(diphenhydramine)*	OK	L2	*
Pepto Bismol Caplets / Chewable Tablets / Original Liquid / Ultra Caplets / Ultra Liquid / Ultra with InstaCool Liquid *(bismuth subsalicylate)*	UNSAFE	L4	
ProVent VertigoX Roll-On Aromatherapy Oils *(herbs)*	UNSAFE	L4	
Sea-Band Acupressure Wrist Bands *(knitted elasticized wristband)*	OK	L1	
Sea-Band Anti-Nausea Ginger Gum *(ginger)*	OK	L1	
Triptone For Motion Sickness Tablets *(dimenhydrinate)*	OK	L2	*

Nasal Preparations

Information Capsules:

 No adverse effects have been reported for **CROMOLYN SODIUM,** and it is regarded as a good alternative nasal spray.

 SODIUM CHLORIDE (SALINE) nasal preparations are considered safe.

		SAFETY LEVEL (PAGE 19)	MONITOR MILK SUPPLY & DRINK EXTRA FLUIDS
4-Way Fast Acting Nasal Decongestant Spray *(phenylephrine)*	OK	L3	*
4-Way Menthol Nasal Decongestant *(menthol / phenylephrine)*	OK	L3	*
Afrin Allergy Sinus Nasal Spray / Original Nasal Spray / Severe Congestion Nasal Spray *(oxymetazoline)*	OK	L3	*
Afrin No Drip Extra Moisturizing Pump Mist Nasal Spray / No Drip Night Pump Mist Nasal Spray / No Drip Original Pump Mist Nasal Spray / No Drip Severe Congestion Pump Mist Nasal Spray / No Drip Sinus Pump Mist Nasal Spray *(oxymetazoline)*	OK	L3	*
Arm & Hammer Simply Saline Nasal Mist Daily Care / Simply Saline Nasal Mist Allergy & Sinus Relief / Simply Saline Nasal Mist Extra Strength / Simply Saline Nasal Mist Nighttime *(sodium chloride)*	OK	L1	
Ayr Allergy & Sinus Hypertonic Saline Nasal Mist / Saline Nasal Mist *(sodium chloride)*	OK	L1	
Ayr Saline Nasal Gel No-Drip Sinus Spray *(aloe / glycerin / sodium chloride)*	OK	L1	
Ayr Saline Nasal Gel With Soothing Aloe *(aloe / dimethicone / glycerin / sodium chloride)*	OK	L1	
Dristan 12 Hour Nasal Spray *(oxymetazoline)*	OK	L3	*
ENTSOL Nasal Gel with Aloe and Vitamin E *(aloe / dimethicone / glycerin / sodium chloride / vitamin E)*	OK	L1	
Flonase Allergy Relief Nasal Spray / Sensimist Allergy Relief Nasal Spray *(fluticasone)*	OK	L3	

* *Additional note applies*   OK *OK to use*   UNSAFE *Do not use*

		SAFETY LEVEL (PAGE 19)	MONITOR MILK SUPPLY & DRINK EXTRA FLUIDS
Mucinex Sinus-Max Severe Nasal Congestion Relief Sinus & Allergy Nasal Spray / Sinus-Max Severe Nasal Congestion Relief Clear & Cool Nasal Spray *(oxymetazoline)*	OK	L3	*
Nasacort Allergy 24 Hour Spray *(triamcinolone)*	OK	L3	
NasalCrom Nasal Allergy Symptom Controller Nasal Spray *(cromolyn sodium)*	OK	L1	
Nasonex 24 Hour Allergy Nasal Spray *(mometasone)*	OK	L3	
NeilMed NasaMist Saline Spray *(sodium bicarbonate / sodium chloride)*	OK	L1	
NeilMed SinuFrin Decongestant Nasal Spray / SinuFrin Plus Decongestant Nasal Spray *(oxymetazoline)*	OK	L3	*
Neo-Synephrine Extra Strength Cold + Allergy Nasal Decongestant Spray / Mild Strength Cold + Allergy Nasal Decongestant Spray / Regular Strength Cold + Allergy Nasal Decongestant Spray *(phenylephrine)*	OK	L3	*
Nose Better Non-Greasy Aromatic Relief Gel *(eucalyptus / menthol)*	OK	L1	
Nostrilla Original Fast Relief Nasal Spray *(oxymetazoline)*	OK	L3	*
Ocean Complete Sinus Rinse *(glycerin / sodium chloride)*	OK	L1	
Ocean Saline Nasal Spray *(sodium chloride)*	OK	L1	
Otrivin Medicated Complete Nasal Care Spray *(xylometazoline)*	OK	L3	*
Pretz Spray Moisturizing Nasal Spray with Yerba Santa *(glycerin / sodium chloride / Yerba santa)*	OK	L1	
Privine Nasal Drops Nasal Decongestant *(naphazoline)*	OK	L3	*
Salinex Daily Care Nasal Spray / Daily Care Nasal Lubricant Spray *(sodium chloride)*	OK	L1	
Similasan Nasal Allergy Relief Preservative Free Homeopathic Nasal Mist *(homeopathic herbs)*	UNSAFE	L4	
Similasan Sinus Relief Preservative Free Homeopathic Nasal Mist *(homeopathic herbs)*	UNSAFE	L4	
Sinarest Nasal Spray *(oxymetazoline)*	OK	L3	*
SinoFresh Nasal & Sinus Care Spray *(eucalyptus oil / peppermint oil / sodium chloride / wintergreen oil)*	OK	L2	

		SAFETY LEVEL (PAGE 19)	MONITOR MILK SUPPLY & DRINK EXTRA FLUIDS
SinuCleanse Nasal Wash *(sodium chloride)*	OK	L1	
Vicks Sinex Nasal Spray For Sinus Relief *(phenylephrine)*	OK	L3	*
Vicks Sinex Saline Ultra Fine Nasal Mist *(sodium chloride)*	OK	L1	
Vicks Sinex Severe Original Nasal Spray / Severe Ultra Fine Mist Nasal Spray / Severe VapoCool Nasal Spray *(oxymetazoline)*	OK	L3	*
Xlear 12 Hour Decongestant Nasal Spray with Oxymetazoline *(oxymetazoline / xylitol)*	OK	L3	*
Xlear Max Saline Nasal Spray with Capsicum *(aloe / capsicum / grapefruit seed extract / sodium chloride / xylitol)*	OK	L2	
Xlear Rescue Xylitol and Saline Nasal Spray *(glycerin / grapefruit seed extract / herbs / sodium chloride / xylitol)*	OK	L1	
Xlear Xylitol and Saline Nasal Spray *(grapefruit seed extract / sodium chloride / xylitol)*	OK	L1	
Zicam Allergy Relief Nasal Swabs with Cooling Menthol *(glycerin / homeopathic herbs / menthol / sodium chloride)*	UNSAFE	L4	
Zicam Allergy Relief No-Drip Liquid Nasal Spray *(glycerin / homeopathic herbs / sodium chloride)*	UNSAFE	L4	
Zicam Cold Remedy Nasal Spray *(eucalyptus / homeopathic herbs / menthol / sodium chloride)*	UNSAFE	L4	
Zicam Extreme Congestion Relief No-Drip Liquid Nasal Spray / Intense Sinus Relief No-Drip Liquid Nasal Spray *(aloe / glycerin / oxymetazoline)*	OK	L3	*
Zicam Intense Sinus Relief No-Drip Liquid Nasal Spray *(aloe / eucalyptus / glycerin / menthol / oxymetazoline)*	OK	L3	*

Ophthalmics (Eye Medications)

		SAFETY LEVEL (PAGE 19)
Advanced Eye Relief Dry Eye Lubricant Eye Drops *(glycerin / propylene glycol)*	OK	L1
Advanced Eye Relief Eye Wash *(irrigating solution)*	OK	L1
Advanced Eye Relief Maximum Redness Eye Drops / Redness Eye Drops *(hypromellose / naphazoline)*	OK	L3
Alaway Eye Itch Relief Eye Drops / Preservative Free Eye Itch Relief Eye Drops *(ketotifen)*	OK	L3
Allersol Ophthalmic Solution *(naphazoline)*	OK	L3
Artelac Nighttime Gel Eye Lubricant *(carbomer / medium chain triglycerides)*	OK	L1
Artelac Rebalance Eye Drops *(hyaluronic acid / PEG-8000)*	OK	L1
Bion Tears Lubricant Eye Drops *(dextran / hypromellose)*	OK	L1
Blink GelTears Lubricating Eye Drops Moderate–Severe / Tears Lubricating Eye Drops Mild–Moderate / Tears Preservative Free Lubricating Eye Drops Mild–Moderate / Triple Care Lubricating Eye Drops Moderate–Severe *(PEG-400)*	OK	L1
Clear Eyes Complete for 7 Symptom Relief Eye Drops *(hypromellose / naphazoline / polysorbate / zinc sulfate)*	OK	L3
Clear Eyes Complete for Sensitive Eyes Eye Drops *(glycerin / phenylephrine)*	OK	L3
Clear Eyes Cooling Comfort Redness Relief Eye Drops / Maximum Redness Relief Eye Drops / Redness Relief Eye Drops *(glycerin / naphazoline)*	OK	L3
Clear Eyes Dry & Itchy Relief Eye Drops *(glycerin)*	OK	L1
Clear Eyes Maximum Itchy Eye Relief Eye Drops *(glycerin / naphazoline / zinc sulfate)*	OK	L3
GenTeal Tears Moderate Liquid Drops *(dextran / glycerin / hypromellose)*	OK	L1
GenTeal Tears Preservative Free Moderate Liquid Drops *(dextran / hypromellose)*	OK	L1
GenTeal Tears Severe Lubricant Eye Gel *(hypromellose)*	OK	L1
GenTeal Tears Severe Night-Time Eye Ointment *(mineral oil / white petrolatum)*	OK	L1

		SAFETY LEVEL (PAGE 19)
Isopto Tears Lubricant Eye Drops (hypromellose)	OK	L1
Just Tears Lubricant Eye Drops (carboxymethylcellulose)	OK	L1
Muro 128 Ointment / Solution (sodium chloride)	OK	L1
Naphcon-A Eye Allergy Relief Eye Drops (naphazoline / pheniramine)	OK	L3
Natural Tears Eye Drops (polyvinyl alcohol / povidone)	OK	L1
Opcon-A Eye Allergy Relief Drops (naphazoline / pheniramine)	OK	L3
Opti-Clear Drops / Solution (tetrahydrazoline)	OK	L3
Opticrom Allergy Eye Drops (cromolyn sodium)	OK	L2
Pataday Once Daily Relief Extra Strength Eye Allergy Itch Relief Drops / Once Daily Relief Eye Allergy Itch Relief Drops / Twice Daily Relief Eye Allergy Itch & Redness Relief Drops (olopatadine)	OK	L2
Refresh Celluvisc Preservative-Free Lubricant Eye Gel (carboxymethylcellulose)	OK	L1
Refresh Classic Preservative-Free Lubricant Eye Drops (polyvinyl alcohol / povidone)	OK	L1
Refresh Lacri-Lube Lubricant Eye Ointment (mineral oil / white petrolatum)	OK	L1
Refresh Liquigel Lubricant Eye Gel (carboxymethylcellulose)	OK	L1
Refresh Optive Lubricant Eye Drops / Optive Preservative-Free Lubricant Eye Drops (carboxymethylcellulose / glycerin)	OK	L1
Refresh Plus Preservative-Free Lubricant Eye Drops / Tears Lubricant Eye Drops (carboxymethylcellulose)	OK	L1
Refresh P.M. Preservative-Free Lubricant Eye Ointment (mineral oil / white petrolatum)	OK	L1
Rohto Cool Relief Redness Relief Eye Drops / Max Strength Maximum Redness Relief Eye Drops (naphazoline / polysorbate 80)	OK	L3
Rohto Digi Eye Digital Eye Strain Eye Drops (hypromellose / tetrahydrozoline)	OK	L3
Rohto Dry Aid Lubricant Eye Drops (povidone / propylene glycol)	OK	L1
Similasan Allergy Eye Relief Homeopathic Eye Drops (homeopathic herbs)	UNSAFE	L4
Similasan Dry Eye Relief Homeopathic Eye Drops (homeopathic herbs)	UNSAFE	L4
Similasan Pink Eye Relief Homeopathic Eye Drops (homeopathic herbs)	UNSAFE	L4

		SAFETY LEVEL (PAGE 19)
Similasan Stye Eye Relief Homeopathic Eye Drops *(homeopathic herbs)*	UNSAFE	L4
Soothe Lubricant Eye Ointment Nighttime Preservative Free Dry Eye Therapy *(mineral oil / white petrolatum)*	OK	L1
Soothe Preservative Free Lubricant Eye Drops *(glycerin / propylene glycol)*	OK	L1
Soothe XP Emollient Lubricant Eye Drops *(light mineral oil / mineral oil)*	OK	L1
Systane Gel Drops Lubricant Eye Gel / Original Lubricant Eye Drops / Original Preservative-Free Lubricant Eye Drops / Ultra Lubricant Eye Drops / Ultra Preservative-Free Lubricant Eye Drops *(PEG-400 / propylene glycol)*	OK	L1
Systane Night Gel Lubricant Eye Gel *(hypromellose)*	OK	L1
Systane Nighttime Lubricant Eye Ointment *(mineral oil / white petrolatum)*	OK	L1
Systane Zaditor Eye Itch Relief Antihistamine Eye Drops *(ketotifen)*	OK	L3
Tears Again Eye Drops / Liquid Gel Drops *(poylvinyl alcohol)*	OK	L1
TheraTears Dry Eye Therapy Lubricant Eye Drops / Dry Eye Therapy Preservative-Free Lubricant Eye Drops / Liquid Gel Nighttime Dry Eye Therapy Lubricant Eye Drops *(carboxymethylcellulose)*	OK	L1
Visine A.C. Itchy Eye Relief Eye Drops *(tetrahydrozoline / zinc sulfate)*	OK	L3
Visine Advanced Redness + Irritation Relief Eye Drops *(dextran / PEG-400 / povidone / tetrahydrozoline)*	OK	L3
Visine Allergy Eye Relief Multi-Action Eye Drops *(naphazoline / pheniramine)*	OK	L3
Visine Dry Eye Relief Tired Eye Drops / Dry Eye Relief Eye Drops *(glycerin / hypromellose / PEG-400)*	OK	L1
Visine Maximum Redness Relief *(glycerin / hypromellose / PEG-400 / tetrahydrozoline)*	OK	L3
Visine Original Redness Relief Eye Drops *(tetrahydrozoline)*	OK	L3
Visine Red Eye Comfort Eye Drops *(glycerin / tetrahydrozoline)*	OK	L3
Visine Red Eye Total Comfort Multi-Symptom Eye Drops *(glycerin / hypromellose / PEG-400 / tetrahydrozoline / zinc sulfate)*	OK	L3

OK *OK to use*   UNSAFE *Do not use*   130   * *Additional note applies*

Oral Hygiene Products (with Mouthwashes and Toothpastes)

Information Capsules:

Oral hygiene products are generally considered compatible with breastfeeding. The ingredients are mostly broken down in the mouth or are not absorbed into the parent's blood to any high degree.

SODIUM FLUORIDE products should be used with care. Look for the amount of sodium fluoride, by weight or by percentage concentration, listed on the product label. Do not use products exceeding 5 mg (10 mL) of sodium fluoride, or a 0.243% concentration of sodium fluoride. Also do not use products exceeding 0.16% concentration of **FLUORIDE ION**. Do not swallow after using.

	SAFETY LEVEL (PAGE 19)	DO NOT USE IF FLUORIDE EXCEEDS 0.243% OR 5 mg (10 mL)	DO NOT SWALLOW AFTER USING
Abreva Cold Sore / Fever Blister Treatment *(docosanol)*	OK L2		
ACT Dry Mouth Lozenges *(glycerin / xylitol)*	OK L1		
Amosan Oral Wound Cleanser Powder Packs *(sodium perborate monohydrate)*	OK L1		
Anbesol Maximum Strength Oral Pain Reliever Gel / Maximum Strength Oral Pain Reliever Liquid *(benzocaine)*	OK L2		
Benzodent Dental Pain Relieving Cream *(benzocaine)*	OK L2		
Biotene Dry Mouth Lozenges *(glycerin / xylitol)*	OK L1		
Biotene Dry Mouth Oral Balance Gel *(bio-enzymes)*	OK L2		
Blister Balm External Analgesic Ointment *(jojoba / menthol / peppermint oil)*	OK L3		
Campho-Phenique Cold Sore Treatment Gel *(camphor / glycerin / phenol)*	UNSAFE L4		

	SAFETY LEVEL (PAGE 19)	DO NOT USE IF FLUORIDE EXCEEDS 0.243% OR 5 mg (10 mL)	DO NOT SWALLOW AFTER USING
Carmex Classic Medicated Lip Balm *(beeswax / camphor / lanolin / menthol / phenol / salicylic acid / white petrolatum)*	OK L1		
Carmex Cold Sore Treatment *(benzocaine / white petrolatum)*	OK L2		
Colgate Peroxyl Mouth Sore Rinse *(hydrogen peroxide)*	OK L1		✳
Crest 3D Whitestrips *(hydrogen peroxide)*	OK L1		
DenTek Canker Relief Advanced Canker Sore Patch *(menthol)*	OK L1		
DenTek Instant Pain Relief Advanced Kit *(benzocaine)*	OK L2		
DenTek Temparin Max Advanced Repair Kit *(eugenol)*	OK L2		
Gly-Oxide Liquid Antiseptic Oral Cleanser *(carbamide peroxide)*	OK L1		
GUM Canker-X Pain Relief Gel *(aloe / castor oil / polyvinylpyrrolidone / propylene glycol)*	OK L3		
GUM Hydral Dry Mouth Relief Oral Gel / Hydral Dry Mouth Relief Oral Rinse *(betaine / polyvinylpyrrolidone / sodium hyaluronate / sorbitol / stevia extract)*	OK L1		✳
GUM Rincinol P.R.N. Mouth Sore Rinse *(aloe / benzalkonium chloride / disodium edetate / glycyrrhetinic acid / propylene glycol / polyvinylpyrrolidone / sodium hyaluronate)*	OK L3		✳
Herpecin-L Lip Balm Stick *(dimethicone)*	OK L2		
Hydrogen peroxide rinse, generic *(hydrogen peroxide)*	OK L1		✳
Kank-A Mouth Pain Liquid *(benzocaine / compound benzoin tincture)*	OK L3		
Kank-A Soft Brush Tooth and Gum Pain Gel *(benzocaine)*	OK L2		
Lip Clear Lysine + Cold Sore Treatment *(lysine / menthol / multiple herbs / vitamins)*	OK L3		
Lubricity Dry Mouth Oral Spray *(potassium sorbate / sodium benzoate / sodium hyaluronate)*	OK L1		

OK *OK to use*   UNSAFE *Do not use*   ✳ *Additional note applies*

		SAFETY LEVEL (PAGE 19)	DO NOT USE IF FLUORIDE EXCEEDS 0.243% OR 5 mg (10 mL)	DO NOT SWALLOW AFTER USING
OraCoat XyliMelts Dry Mouth Stick-On Melts for Moisturizing *(acacia gum / calcium carbonate / cellulose gum / magnesium stearate / sodium bicarbonate)*	OK	L3		
Orajel 3X Medicated for All Mouth Sores Gel *(benzocaine / menthol / zinc chloride)*	OK	L3		
Orajel Antiseptic Mouth Sore Rinse *(hydrogen peroxide / menthol)*	OK	L1		✱
Orajel Cold Sore MoistureLock Cream *(allantoin / benzocaine / camphor / dimethicone / menthol / white petrolatum)*	OK	L2		
Orajel Cold Sore Touch-Free Liquid Balm *(benzalkonium chloride / benzocaine)*	OK	L3		
Orajel Medicated for Toothache Gel *(benzocaine)*	OK	L2		
Red Cross Toothache Medication *(eugenol / sesame oil)*	OK	L2		
Releev 1 Day Cold Sore Symptom Treatment *(benzalkonium chloride)*	OK	L3		
Rembrandt Whitening Strips *(hydrogen peroxide)*	OK	L1		
TheraBreath Dry Mouth Lozenges *(citric acid / sorbitol / spilanthes acmella flower extract / zinc / zinc gluconate)*	OK	L1		
Zilactin-B 6 Hour Canker & Mouth Sore Relief Gel / Long Lasting Mouth Sore Gel *(benzocaine / boric acid / salicylic acid)*	OK	L2		
Zilactin Early Relief Cold Sore Gel / Tooth and Gum Instant Pain Reliever *(benzyl alcohol / boric acid / salicylic acid)*	OK	L2		

Mouthwashes

		SAFETY LEVEL (PAGE 19)	DO NOT USE IF FLUORIDE EXCEEDS 0.243% OR 5 mg (10 mL)	DO NOT SWALLOW AFTER USING
ACT Anticavity Mouthwash / Restoring Mouthwash / Total Care Mouthwash *(cetylpyridinium chloride / poloxamer 407 / propylene glycol / sodium fluoride)*	OK	L2	✱	✱
ACT Dry Mouth Mouthwash *(betaine / cetylpyridinium chloride / ginger / glycerin / poloxamer 407 / propylene glycol / sorbitol / xylitol)*	OK	L3		✱

		SAFETY LEVEL (PAGE 19)	DO NOT USE IF FLUORIDE EXCEEDS 0.243% OR 5 mg (10 mL)	DO NOT SWALLOW AFTER USING
ACT Whitening Mouthwash *(hydrogen peroxide / poloxamer 407 / propylene glycol / sodium fluoride)*	OK	L2	*	*
Anti-plaque dental rinse, generic *(benzoic acid / ethyl alcohol / glycerin / sorbitol / tetrasodium pyrophosphate)*	OK	L2		*
Biotene Dry Mouth Gentle Oral Rinse / Dry Mouth Oral Rinse *(glycerin / hydroxyethylcellulose / poloxamer 407 / propylene glycol / sorbitol / xylitol)*	OK	L1		*
Cepacol Antibacterial Mouthwash *(cetylpyridinium chloride / glycerin / ethyl alcohol)*	OK	L1		*
Close-Up Mouthwash *(eugenol / glycerin / poloxamer 407 / sodium fluoride / sorbitol)*	OK	L2	*	*
CloSYS Sensitive Mouthwash *(chlorine dioxide / trisodium phosphate)*	OK	L2		*
Colgate Fluorigard Fluoride Rinse *(cetylpyridinium chloride / sodium fluoride / sodium phosphate / sorbitol)*	OK	L2	*	*
Colgate Phos Flur Ortho Defense Fluoride Rinse *(phosphoric acid / sodium fluoride / sodium phosphate / sorbitol)*	OK	L2	*	*
Crest 3D White Brilliance Mouthwash / Glamorous White Mouthwash *(glycerin / hydrogen peroxide / poloxamer 407 / propylene glycol / sodium hexametaphosphate)*	OK	L1		*
Crest Pro-Health Advanced Extra Whitening Mouthwash *(glycerin / hydrogen peroxide / poloxamer 407 / sodium fluoride)*	OK	L2	*	*
Crest Pro-Health Advanced Mouthwash *(cetylpyridinium chloride / glycerin / poloxamer 407 / sodium fluoride)*	OK	L2	*	*
Listerine Cool Mint Antiseptic Mouthwash *(ethyl alcohol / poloxamer 407 / sorbitol / thymol)*	OK	L2		*
Listerine Total Care Anticavity Mouthwash *(poloxamer 407 / sodium fluoride / sorbitol / thymol)*	OK	L2	*	*
PLAX Prebrushing Dental Rinse *(benzoic acid / ethyl alcohol / poloxamer 407 / sorbitol / tetrasodium pyrophosphate)*	OK	L2		*

		SAFETY LEVEL (PAGE 19)	DO NOT USE IF FLUORIDE EXCEEDS 0.243% OR 5 mg (10 mL)	DO NOT SWALLOW AFTER USING
Scope Classic Mouthwash *(cetylpyridinium chloride / ethyl alcohol / glycerin)*	OK	L1		*
Smart Mouth Original Zinc Activated Breath Rinse *(glycerin / poloxamer 407 / sodium chloride / sodium chlorite / zinc chloride)*	OK	L3		*
TheraBreath Fresh Breath Oral Rinse *(peppermint / sodium chlorite)*	OK	L2		*
Tom's of Maine Whole Care Mouthwash *(aloe / glycerin / sodium fluoride / sorbitol)*	OK	L2	*	*

Toothpastes

Aim Anticavity Toothpaste *(sodium fluoride)*	OK	L2	*	*
Aquafresh Cavity Protection Toothpaste *(sodium fluoride)*	OK	L2	*	*
Aquafresh Sensitive Toothpaste *(potassium nitrate / sodium fluoride)*	OK	L2	*	*
Arm & Hammer Advance White Baking Soda and Peroxide Toothpaste / Advance White Extreme Whitening Toothpaste / PeroxiCare Toothpaste *(baking soda / sodium carbonate peroxide / sodium fluoride)*	OK	L2	*	*
Arm & Hammer Complete Care Toothpaste / Dental Care Toothpaste *(baking soda / sodium fluoride)*	OK	L2	*	*
Arm & Hammer Sensitive Toothpaste *(baking soda / potassium nitrate / sodium fluoride)*	OK	L2	*	*
Burt's Bees Charcoal + Whitening Fluoride Toothpaste *(activated charcoal / cocamidopropyl betaine / glycerin / hydrated silica / sodium fluoride / stevia extract)*	OK	L3	*	*
Burt's Bees Purely White Zen Peppermint Fluoride-Free Toothpaste *(cocamidopropyl betaine / glycerin / hydrated silica / stevia extract)*	OK	L3		*
Close-Up Triple Fresh Formula Toothpaste *(cocamidopropyl betaine / eugenol / hydrated silica / sodium fluoride / tea tree extract / zinc sulfate)*	OK	L2	*	*

---

* *Additional note applies*   135   OK *OK to use*   UNSAFE *Do not use*

		SAFETY LEVEL (PAGE 19)	DO NOT USE IF FLUORIDE EXCEEDS 0.243% OR 5 mg (10 mL)	DO NOT SWALLOW AFTER USING
Colgate Sensitive Toothpastes with sodium fluoride (hydrated silica / poloxamer 407 / potassium nitrate / sodium fluoride / sorbitol)	OK	L2	*	*
Colgate Sensitive Toothpastes with stannous fluoride (cocamidopropyl betaine / hydrated silica / stannous fluoride)	OK	L1	*	*
Colgate Toothpastes with sodium fluoride (cocamidopropyl betaine / hydrated silica / sodium fluoride / sorbitol)	OK	L2	*	*
Colgate Toothpastes with stannous fluoride (cocamidopropyl betaine / glycerin / hydrated silica / sorbitol / stannous fluoride)	OK	L1	*	*
Colgate Whitening Toothpastes with baking soda (baking soda / hydrated silica / sodium monofluorophosphate)	OK	L2	*	*
Colgate Whitening Toothpastes with hydrogen peroxide (hydrogen peroxide / sodium monofluorophosphate)	OK	L2	*	*
Colgate Whitening Toothpastes with sodium fluoride (cocamidopropyl betaine / hydrated silica / sodium fluoride / sorbitol)	OK	L2	*	*
Colgate Whitening Toothpastes with stannous fluoride (cocamidopropyl betaine / hydrated silica / stannous fluoride)	OK	L1	*	*
Crest 3D White Toothpaste with hydrogen peroxide (hydrogen peroxide / sodium monofluorophosphate)	OK	L2	*	*
Crest 3D White Toothpastes with sodium fluoride and disodium pyrophosphate (disodium pyrophosphate / hydrated silica / sodium fluoride / sorbitol)	OK	L2	*	*
Crest 3D White Toothpastes with sodium fluoride and sodium hexametaphosphate (sodium fluoride / hydrated silica / sodium hexametaphosphate)	OK	L2	*	*
Crest Baking Soda & Peroxide Whitening Toothpaste (baking soda / hydrated silica / peroxide / poloxamer 407 / propylene glycol / sodium fluoride / sorbitol)	OK	L2	*	*

		SAFETY LEVEL (PAGE 19)	DO NOT USE IF FLUORIDE EXCEEDS 0.243% OR 5 mg (10 mL)	DO NOT SWALLOW AFTER USING
Crest Pro-Health Advanced Toothpastes with stannous fluoride and sodium hexametaphosphate *(hydrated silica / propylene glycol / sodium hexametaphosphate / stannous fluoride)*	OK	L1	✳	✳
Crest Pro-Health Whitening Toothpastes with stannous fluoride *(hydrated silica / sorbitol / stannous fluoride)*	OK	L1	✳	✳
Crest Sensitive Toothpastes with sodium fluoride and potassium nitrate *(cetylpyridinium chloride / hydrated silica / potassium nitrate / sodium fluoride / sorbitol)*	OK	L2	✳	✳
Crest Whitening Toothpastes with sodium fluoride *(disodium pyrophosphate / sodium fluoride / sorbitol / hydrated silica)*	OK	L2	✳	✳
Parodontax Active Gum Repair Toothpaste / Complete Protection Toothpaste / Complete Protection Whitening Toothpaste / Toothpaste / Whitening Toothpaste *(cocamidopropyl betaine / hydrated silica / pentasodium triphosphate / stannous fluoride)*	OK	L1	✳	✳
Pepsodent Charcoal White Toothpaste *(activated charcoal / hydrated silica / mica / perlite / sodium fluoride / sorbitol / zinc citrate)*	OK	L2	✳	✳
Pepsodent Germicheck Toothpaste *(calcium carbonate / hydrated silica / sodium monofluorophosphate / sorbitol)*	OK	L2	✳	✳
Pepsodent Sensitive Expert Toothpaste *(hydrated silica / hydroxyapatite / sodium monofluorophosphate / sorbitol / zinc citrate)*	OK	L2	✳	✳
Rembrandt Deeply White + Peroxide Toothpaste *(calcium pyrophosphate / hydrogen peroxide / sodium monofluorophosphate)*	OK	L1	✳	✳
Rembrandt Intense Stain Toothpaste *(cocamidopropyl betaine / hydrated silica / sodium fluoride / sorbitol / tetrasodium pyrophosphate)*	OK	L2	✳	✳
Sensodyne Natural White Toothpastes *(activated charcoal / cocamidopropyl betaine / hydrated silica / potassium nitrate / sodium fluoride / sorbitol)*	OK	L2	✳	✳

✳ *Additional note applies*

OK *OK to use*   UNSAFE *Do not use*

	Safety Level	Safety Level (page 19)	DO NOT USE IF FLUORIDE EXCEEDS 0.243% OR 5 mg (10 mL)	DO NOT SWALLOW AFTER USING
Sensodyne Nourish Toothpastes *(aloe / cocamidopropyl betaine / coconut oil / glycerin / hydrated silica / potassium nitrate / sodium fluoride / sorbitol)*	OK	L2	*	*
Sensodyne Pronamel Toothpastes *(cocamidopropyl betaine / hydrated silica / potassium nitrate / sodium fluoride / sodium hydroxide / sorbitol)*	OK	L2	*	*
Sensodyne Toothpastes with potassium nitrate and sodium fluoride *(cocamidopropyl betaine / hydrated silica / pentasodium triphosphate / potassium nitrate / sodium fluoride)*	OK	L2	*	*
Sensodyne Toothpastes with stannous fluoride *(cocamidopropyl betaine / hydrated silica / pentasodium triphosphate / stannous fluoride)*	OK	L1	*	*
Tom's of Maine Antiplaque and Whitening Toothpaste *(calcium carbonate / glycerin / hydrated silica / zinc citrate)*	OK	L1		*
Tom's of Maine Luminous White Toothpaste / Simply White Toothpaste *(glycerin / hydrated silica / sodium fluoride / sorbitol)*	OK	L2	*	*
Tom's of Maine Rapid Relief Sensitive Toothpaste *(arginine bicarbonate / calcium carbonate / hydrated silica / sorbitol)*	OK	L1		*
Tom's of Maine Whole Care Toothpaste *(calcium carbonate / glyerin / hydrated silica / sodium monofluorophosphate / zinc citrate)*	OK	L2	*	*

Otics (Ear Medications)

		SAFETY LEVEL (PAGE 19)
Auro-Dri Ear Drying Aid *(glycerin / isopropyl alcohol)*	OK	L1
Debrox Earwax Removal Aid Drops *(carbamide peroxide)*	OK	L1
EARWAX MD Earwax Dissolving Drops *(glycerin)*	OK	L1
Hyland's Earache Drops *(glycerin / homeopathic herbs)*	OK	L3
Mack's Dry-n-Clear Ear Drying Aid *(glycerin / isopropyl alcohol)*	OK	L1
Murine Ear Wax Removal Kit / Carbamide Peroxide Ear Wax Removal Aid *(carbamide peroxide)*	OK	L1
NeilMed ClearCanal Earwax Removal Complete Kit *(carbamide peroxide)*	OK	L1
Similasan Earache Relief Ear Drops / Ear Wax Relief Ear Drops *(glycerin / homeopathic herbs)*	OK	L3
Swim Ear Drying Aid *(glycerin / isopropyl alcohol)*	OK	L1
The Relief Products (TRP) Ring Relief Ear Drops / Tablets *(glycerin / homeopathic herbs)*	OK	L3

Moisturizers and Skin Lubricants (with Scar and Stretch Mark Therapy Products)

For each product below, the primary hydrating, smoothing, and protecting ingredients are listed. Note that individual products may also contain acids, alcohols, animal by-products, dyes, emulsifiers, enzymes, fillers, food products, fragrances, herbs, minerals, moisturizers, oils, preservatives, stabilizers, sunscreens, and/or water. Always check the full ingredients listed on the label to determine if you are allergic to any of the ingredients or if they are suitable for your skin type.

Information Capsules:

 Ingredients in moisturizers are usually compatible with breastfeeding because they are applied topically in low concentrations.

 For **ALL PRODUCTS** listed below, if applied to the nipple or areola, clean the area with warm water and mild soap before breastfeeding.

		SAFETY LEVEL (PAGE 19)
AmLactin Daily Moisturizing Lotion *(dimethicone / glycerin / lactic acid / mineral oil)*	OK	L1
AmLactin Foot Repair Cream *(glycerin / lactic acid / mineral oil / petrolatum)*	OK	L1
AmLactin Rapid Relief Restoring Lotion *(ceramides / dimethicone / glycerin / lactic acid / mineral oil / petrolatum)*	OK	L1
Ammonium lactate lotion, generic *(ammonium lactate)*	OK	L1
A+D Original Ointment *(cod liver oil / lanolin / petrolatum / vitamin A / vitamin D)*	OK	L1
Aqua Care Lotion *(lactic acid / mineral oil / petrolatum / urea)*	OK	L1
Aquaphor Healing Ointment *(ceresin / glycerin / lanolin / mineral oil / petrolatum)*	OK	L1

		SAFETY LEVEL (PAGE 19)
Australian Gold Soothing Aloe Vera Gel *(aloe)*	OK	L1
Aveeno Creamy Oil Moisturizer *(glycerin / oat flour / sweet almond oil)*	OK	L1
Aveeno Daily Moisturizing Body Lotion *(dimethicone / glycerin / oat kernel flour / petrolatum)*	OK	L1
Aveeno Daily Moisturizing Face Cream / Daily Moisturizing Sheer Hydration Body Lotion *(dimethicone / glycerin / oat kernel flour)*	OK	L1
Aveeno Positively Radiant Daily Moisturizer with SPF 15 / Ultra-Calming Daily Moisturizer with SPF 15 *(dimethicone / glycerin)*	OK	L1
Aveeno Skin Relief Moisture Repair Cream / Skin Relief Moisturizing Lotion / Skin Relief Overnight Cream *(dimethicone / glycerin / oat kernel flour / petrolatum / shea butter)*	OK	L1
Aveeno Soothing Oatmeal Bath Treatment *(colloidal oatmeal)*	OK	L1
Banana Boat Soothing Aloe After Sun Gel *(aloe / glycerin)*	OK	L1
Bio-Oil Skincare Oil *(mineral oil / multiple natural oils)*	OK	L1
CeraVe AM Facial Moisturizing Lotion with Sunscreen *(ceramides / dimethicone / glycerin / hyaluronic acid)*	OK	L1
CeraVe Daily Moisturizing Lotion *(ceramides / dimethicone / hyaluronic acid)*	OK	L1
CeraVe Diabetics' Dry Skin Relief Hand & Foot Cream *(bilberry extract / ceramides / glycerin / urea)*	OK	L1
CeraVe Moisturizing Cream *(ceramides / dimethicone / hyaluronic acid / petrolatum)*	OK	L1
CeraVe SA Cream for Rough & Bumpy Skin *(ammonium lactate / ceramides / corn oil / dimethicone / glycerin / mineral oil / hyaluronic acid / salicylic acid)*	OK	L1
Cetaphil Advanced Relief Cream *(dimethicone / glycerin / safflower oil / shea butter)*	OK	L1
Cetaphil Cracked Skin Repair Balm *(dimethicone / glycerin / shea butter)*	OK	L1
Cetaphil Daily Facial Moisturizer SPF 15 *(glycerin)*	OK	L1
Cetaphil Daily Oil-Free Hydrating Lotion *(glycerin / hyaluronic acid)*	OK	L1
Cetaphil Moisturizing Cream *(dimethicone / glycerin / petrolatum / sunflower oil / sweet almond oil)*	OK	L1
Cetaphil Moisturizing Lotion *(avocado oil / dimethicone / glycerin / sunflower seed oil)*	OK	L1

		SAFETY LEVEL (PAGE 19)
Cetaphil Rough & Bumpy Daily Smoothing Moisturizer *(dimethicone / glycerin / sweet almond oil / urea)*	OK	L1
Cocoa butter stick, generic *(cocoa butter)*	OK	L1
Curél Daily Healing Original Lotion *(dimethicone / eucalyptus / glycerin / petrolatum / shea butter)*	OK	L1
Curél Foot Therapy Cream *(dimethicone / glycerin / paraffin / olive oil / petrolatum / shea butter / urea)*	OK	L1
Curél Fragrance Free Original Lotion *(dimethicone / eucalyptus / glycerin / petrolatum)*	OK	L1
Curél Ultra Healing Original Lotion *(dimethicone / eucalyptus / glycerin / oat kernel extract / petrolatum / shea butter)*	OK	L1
Dove Body Love Everyday Care Body Lotion *(dimethicone / glycerin / mineral oil / sunflower oil)*	OK	L1
Dove Body Love Intense Care Body Lotion *(dimethicone / glycerin / mineral oil / petrolatum / sunflower oil)*	OK	L1
Dove Body Love Sensitive Care Body Lotion *(dimethicone / glycerin / sunflower oil / petrolatum)*	OK	L1
Dr. Nice's Moisturizing Gel *(peppermint oil / poloxamer 407)*	OK	L1
Dr. Scholl's Ultra Hydrating Foot Cream *(aloe / dimethicone / petrolatum / urea)*	OK	L1
Duke Cannon Dry Ice Body Spray Powder *(aloe / eucalyptus / menthol / peppermint oil / baking soda / zinc oxide)*	OK	L1
Duke Cannon Grunt Foot and Boot Powder Spray *(activated charcoal / calamine / eucalyptus oil / menthol)*	OK	L3
Dynarex Vitamins A&D Ointment *(lanolin / mineral oil / petrolatum / vitamin A / vitamin D)*	OK	L1
Eucerin Advanced Repair Foot Cream / Advanced Repair Hand Cream *(ceramides / dimethicone / glycerin / lactic acid / sunflower oil / urea)*	OK	L1
Eucerin Advanced Repair Lotion *(ceramides / glycerin / lactic acid / shea butter / urea)*	OK	L1
Eucerin Daily Hydration Lotion *(dimethicone / glycerin / petrolatum / sunflower oil)*	OK	L1
Eucerin Daily Protection Face Lotion SPF 30 *(castor oil / dimethicone / glycerin / lactic acid)*	OK	L1

		SAFETY LEVEL (PAGE 19)
Eucerin Intensive Repair Lotion *(castor oil / dimethicone / glycerin / lactic acid / lanolin / mineral oil / urea)*	OK	L1
Eucerin Original Healing Cream *(lanolin / mineral oil / petrolatum)*	OK	L1
Eucerin Original Healing Lotion *(lanolin / mineral oil)*	OK	L1
Eucerin Skin Calming Cream *(colloidal oatmeal / dimethicone / glycerin / mineral oil / piroctone olamine)*	OK	L1
Flexitol Heel Balm *(allantoin / aloe / glycolic acid / lanolin / mineral oil / shea butter / tea tree oil / urea)*	OK	L1
Gold Bond Healing Foot Cream *(aloe / dimethicone / glycerin / lactic acid / petrolatum / urea)*	OK	L1
Gold Bond Healing Hydrating Cream *(aloe / dimethicone / glycerin / petrolatum)*	OK	L1
Gold Bond Medicated Diabetics' Dry Skin Relief Foot Cream *(allantoin / aloe / dimethicone / glycerin / shea butter / white petrolatum)*	OK	L1
Gold Bond Overnight Deep Moisturizing Lotion *(aloe / ceramides / coconut oil / dimethicone / glycerin / petrolatum / shea butter / urea)*	OK	L1
Gold Bond Ultimate Comfort Body Powder *(aloe / corn starch / baking soda)*	OK	L1
Hawaiian Tropic After Sun Body Butter *(avocado oil / cocoa butter / coconut oil / glycerin / mango butter / shea butter)*	OK	L1
Hawaiian Tropic Body Lotion and Moisturizer After Sun / Sheer Touch Lotion Sunscreen *(aloe / cocoa butter / glycerin / petrolatum / shea butter)*	OK	L1
Jergens Daily Moisture Dry Skin Moisturizer *(citrus extracts / dimethicone / glycerin / mineral oil)*	OK	L1
Jergens Instant Sunless Tanning Moisturizer + Bronzer *(coconut oil / corn starch / dihydroxyacetone / dimethicone / glycerin / mineral oil / petrolatum)*	OK	L1
Jergens Natural Glow Daily Moisturizer *(avocado oil / coconut oil / corn starch / dihydroxyacetone / dimethicone / glycerin / mineral oil / oat extract / olive oil / petrolatum)*	OK	L1
Jergens Original Scent Dry Skin Lotion *(dimethicone / glycerin / lanolin oil)*	OK	L1
Jergens Skin Firming and Toning Moisturizer *(caffeine / coconut water / dimethicone / glycerin / mineral oil / petrolatum)*	OK	L1
Jergens Ultra Healing Extra Dry Skin Moisturizer *(allantoin / dimethicone / glycerin / petrolatum)*	OK	L1

		SAFETY LEVEL (PAGE 19)
Jergens Wet Skin Moisturizer *(glycerin / hyaluronic acid / mineral oil)*	OK	L1
Johnson's Aloe and Vitamin E Powder *(aloe / corn starch / vitamin E)*	OK	L1
Johnson's Baby Oil *(mineral oil)*	OK	L1
Kerasal Intensive Foot Repair Cream *(glycerin / salicylic acid / urea)*	OK	L1
Keri Daily Moisture Original Lotion *(aloe / glycerin / mineral oil / sunflower oil)*	OK	L1
Keri Moisture Rich Shower and Bath Oil *(lanolin oil / mineral oil)*	OK	L1
Keri Nourishing Shea Butter Lotion *(aloe / glycerin / mineral oil / shea butter / sunflower oil)*	OK	L1
La Roche-Posay Hyalu B5 Pure Hyaluronic Acid Serum *(dimethicone / glycerin / hyaluronic acid)*	OK	L1
La Roche-Posay Toleriane Ultra Soothing Repair Moisturizer *(dimethicone / glycerin / neurosensine / shea butter)*	OK	L1
La Roche-Posay Triple Repair Moisturizing Cream *(ceramides / dimethicone / glycerin / shea butter)*	OK	L1
La Roche-Posay Vitamin C Serum *(dimethicone / glycerin / hyaluronic acid / salicylic acid / vitamin C)*	OK	L1
Lanolin hydrous ointment, generic *(lanolin)*	OK	L1
Lubriderm Advanced Therapy Lotion / Daily Moisture Lotion *(dimethicone / glycerin / mineral oil)*	OK	L1
Lubriderm Advanced Therapy Moisturizing Cream *(dimethicone / glycerin / linseed oil / mineral oil / petrolatum / shea butter)*	OK	L1
Lubriderm Daily Moisture Lotion with Sunscreen *(glycerin)*	OK	L1
Lubriderm Intense Skin Repair Lotion *(glycerin / mineral oil / petrolatum / shea butter)*	OK	L1
Mederma Quick Dry Oil *(multiple natural oils)*	OK	L1
Mineral oil, generic *(mineral oil)*	OK	L1
Neutrogena Deep Moisture Day Cream with Sunscreen *(dimethicone / glycerin / shea butter)*	OK	L1
Neutrogena Hydro Boost Body Gel Cream *(dimethicone / glycerin / hyaluronic acid / petrolatum)*	OK	L1
Neutrogena Norwegian Formula Hand Cream *(glycerin)*	OK	L1

		SAFETY LEVEL (PAGE 19)
Nivea Creme *(glycerin / lanolin / mineral oil / paraffin / petrolatum)*	OK	L1
Nivea Essentially Enriched Body Lotion *(glycerin / mineral oil / petrolatum / sweet almond oil)*	OK	L1
Nivea Original Moisture Body Lotion *(glycerin / lanolin / mineral oil)*	OK	L1
Nivea Smooth Sensation Body Lotion *(dimethicone / glycerin / lanolin / mineral oil)*	OK	L1
O'Keeffe's for Healthy Feet Cream / Working Hands Cream *(allantoin / dimethicone / glycerin / paraffin / urea)*	OK	L1
Olay Regenerist Micro Sculpting Cream *(dimethicone / glycerin / hyaluronic acid / peptides / vitamins)*	OK	L1
Olay Regenerist Vitamin C + Peptide24 Moisturizer *(dimethicone / glycerin / lactic acid / peptides / vitamin C)*	OK	L1
Olay Retinol24 Night Moisturizer *(dimethicone / glycerin / retinol)*	OK	L1
Olay Total Effects 7 in One Moisturizer *(dimethicone / glycerin / green tea extract / vitamins)*	OK	L1
Palmer's Cocoa Butter Formula Daily Skin Therapy Lotion *(cocoa butter / coconut oil / dimethicone / glycerin / mineral oil / petrolatum / sunflower oil)*	OK	L1
Palmer's Cocoa Butter Formula Skin Therapy Oil *(canola oil / cocoa butter / rosehip oil / sesame oil)*	OK	L1
Petroleum jelly, generic *(white petrolatum)*	OK	L1
pHisoderm Clean Sensitive Skin Cream Cleanser *(aloe / glycerin / sunflower oil)*	OK	L1
Pond's Cold Cream Cleanser *(beeswax / ceresin / mineral oil)*	OK	L1
Pond's Dry Skin Cream Moisturizer *(beeswax / ceresin / glycerin / mineral oil / petrolatum)*	OK	L1
Queen Helene Cocoa Butter Crème *(beeswax / cocoa butter / mineral oil / paraffin)*	OK	L1
SheaMoisture Ultra Hydration 100% Raw Shea Butter *(shea butter)*	OK	L1
SunBurnt Daily After-Sun Lotion *(aloe / coconut oil / dimethicone / glycerin / shea butter)*	OK	L1
Tucks Medicated Cooling Pads *(glycerin / witch hazel)*	OK	L1
Vanicream Moisturizing Cream / Moisturizing Lotion *(petrolatum)*	OK	L1

✳ *Additional note applies*   145   OK *OK to use*   UNSAFE *Do not use*

		SAFETY LEVEL (PAGE 19)
Vanicream Moisturizing Ointment *(dimethicone / hydrogenated polydecene)*	OK	L1
Vaseline Clinical Care Dry Hands Rescue *(carnauba wax / dimethicone / glycerin / petrolatum)*	OK	L1
Vaseline Clinical Care Extremely Dry Skin Rescue Lotion *(dimethicone / glycerin / mineral oil / petrolatum)*	OK	L1
Vaseline Intensive Care Advanced Repair Lotion *(dimethicone / glycerin / mineral oil / petrolatum / shea butter / sunflower oil)*	OK	L1
Vaseline Intensive Care Cocoa Radiant Lotion *(cocoa butter / coconut oil / dimethicone / glycerin / petrolatum / sunflower oil)*	OK	L1
Vaseline Intensive Care Deep Moisture Jelly Cream *(glycerin / white petrolatum)*	OK	L1
Vaseline Intensive Care Healthy Hands Stronger Nails Lotion *(dimethicone / glycerin / mineral oil)*	OK	L1
Vaseline Intensive Care Soothing Hydration Lotion *(aloe / dimethicone / glycerin / petrolatum / sunflower oil)*	OK	L1
Vaseline Original Healing Jelly *(white petrolatum)*	OK	L1
Vitamins A&D ointment, generic *(cod liver oil / lanolin / vitamin A / vitamin D)*	OK	L1
Zim's Crack Creme *(Arnica montana / glycerin / myrcia oil)*	OK	L1
Zinc oxide ointment, generic *(zinc oxide)*	OK	L1

Scar and Stretch Mark Therapy Products

Cicatricure Face & Body Scar Gel *(allantoin / aloe / glycerin / onion extract / urea)*	OK	L1
Mederma Advanced Scar Gel *(allantoin / onion extract)*	OK	L1
Mederma Stretch Marks Therapy Cream *(dimethicone / glycerin / onion extract)*	OK	L1
Mustela Stretch Marks Cream *(avocado oil / glycerin / passion fruit oil / shea butter / witch hazel)*	OK	L1
Mustela Stretch Marks Oil *(avocado oil / passion fruit oil / sunflower oil)*	OK	L1
New Skin Scar Fade Gel *(dimethicone)*	OK	L1

		SAFETY LEVEL (PAGE 19)
Palmer's Cocoa Butter Formula Massage Lotion for Stretch Marks *(cocoa butter / cocoa extract / coconut oil / dimethicone / glycerin / petrolatum / shea butter / sunflower oil / sweet almond oil)*	OK	L1
PreferOn Intensive Scar Management Stick *(dimethicone / onion extract / urea)*	OK	L1
ScarAway Silicone Scar Gel *(silicone)*	OK	L1
Scarguard Repair Liquid *(hydrocortisone / silicone)*	OK	L1

Pediculosis (Lice) Treatments

		SAFETY LEVEL (PAGE 19)
CVS Health Lice Killing Shampoo Maximum Strength *(piperonyl butoxide / pyrethrum extract)*	OK	L2
Lice MD Lice and Egg Removal Liquid Gel Kit *(dimethicone)*	OK	L1
Lice Shield Leave-In Spray / Shampoo and Conditioner in 1 *(cedar oil / citronella oil / geraniol / lemongrass oil / rosemary oil)*	OK	L1
Licefreee! Everyday Shampoo / Gel / Spray *(sodium chloride)*	OK	L3
LiceGuard No-Nit Kit *(benzisothiazolinone / methylisothiazolinone)*	OK	L3
Nix Lice Killing Creme Rinse *(permethrin)*	OK	L2
Permethrin lotion, generic *(permethrin)*	OK	L2
RID Lice Killing Shampoo *(piperonyl butoxide / pyrethrum extract)*	OK	L2
RID Super MAX Solution *(acrylate copolymer / hydrogenated didecene / hydrogenated polydecene / sunflower oil)*	OK	L1
Rite Aid Lice Shampoo *(piperonyl butoxide / pyrethrum extract)*	OK	L2

Pinworm Treatments

Information Capsules:

 Pinworm treatment medications (**PYRANTEL PAMOATE**) are not absorbed readily from the gastrointestinal tract, so only very small amounts of these drugs appear in breastmilk. They are considered compatible with breastfeeding.

		SAFETY LEVEL (PAGE 19)
CVS Health Pinworm Treatment *(pyrantel pamoate)*	OK	L3
Reese's Pinworm Treatment Suspension *(pyrantel pamoate)*	OK	L3
Walgreens Pinworm Medicine *(pyrantel pamoate)*	OK	L3

Sleep Aid Preparations

	SAFETY LEVEL (P. 19)	MONITOR INFANT FOR DROWS-INESS	LOOK FOR ALTERNATIVE THAT DOES NOT COMBINE INGREDIENTS	DO NOT EXCEED MELATONIN DOSE OF 3 mg PER DAY
Advil PM Caplets / Liqui-Gels *(diphenhydramine / ibuprofen)*	OK L2	*	*	
Aleve PM *(diphenhydramine / naproxen)*	OK L3	*	*	
Benadryl Capsules *(diphenhydramine)*	OK L2	*		
Dormin Capsules *(diphenhydramine)*	OK L2	*		
Excedrin PM Caplets / Tablets *(acetaminophen / aspirin / diphenhydramine)*	UNSAFE L4			
Goody's PM Powders *(acetaminophen / diphenhydramine)*	OK L2	*	*	
Hyland's Calms Forté Tablets *(homeopathic herbs)*	UNSAFE L4			
Hyland's Rest Tablets *(homeopathic herbs)*	UNSAFE L4			
Hyland's Restful Legs PM Tablets *(homeopathic herbs)*	UNSAFE L4			
Legatrin PM Caplets *(acetaminophen / diphenhydramine)*	OK L2	*	*	
Major Mapap PM Extra Strength Caplets *(acetaminophen / diphenhydramine)*	OK L2	*	*	
Melatonin pills / tablets / gummies, generic *(melatonin - 1 mg, 2 mg, 2.5 mg, or 3 mg)*	OK L2			*
Melatonin pills / tablets / gummies, generic *(melatonin - 4 mg, 5 mg, or 10 mg)*	UNSAFE L3			
MidNite Sleep Health Supplement Chewable Tablets *(chamomile / lavender / lemon / melatonin - 1.5 mg)*	OK L2	*		*
Motrin PM Caplets *(diphenhydramine / ibuprofen)*	OK L2	*	*	

		SAFETY LEVEL (P. 19)	MONITOR INFANT FOR DROWS-INESS	LOOK FOR ALTERNATIVE THAT DOES NOT COMBINE INGREDIENTS	DO NOT EXCEED MELATONIN DOSE OF 3 mg PER DAY
Natrol 3 a.m. Melatonin Fast Dissolve Tablets / Melatonin Calm Sleep Fast Dissolve Tablets *(L-theanine / melatonin - 3 mg or 6 mg)*	OK	L3			*
Natrol Liquid Melatonin / Melatonin Fast Dissolve Tablets / Melatonin Gummies *(melatonin - 1 mg, 2.5 mg, 3 mg, 5 mg, or 10 mg)*	OK	L3			*
Natrol Melatonin Advanced Maximum Strength Time Release Tablets / Melatonin Tablets *(calcium / melatonin - 1 mg, 3 mg, 5 mg, or 10 mg / vitamin B6)*	OK	L3			*
Natrol Melatonin Time Release Tablets *(melatonin - 1 mg, 3 mg, or 5 mg / vitamin B6)*	OK	L3			*
Nature Made Melatonin Extended Release Tablets / Melatonin Tablets *(calcium / melatonin - 3 mg, 4 mg, 5 mg, 10 mg)*	OK	L3			*
Nature Made Melatonin Gummies *(melatonin - 2.5 mg, 5 mg, or 10 mg)*	OK	L3			*
Nature's Bounty Dual Spectrum Melatonin Bi-Layer Tablets / Melatonin Capsules / Melatonin Rapid Release Softgels / Melatonin Tablets / Sleep Gummies *(melatonin - 1 mg, 3 mg, 5 mg, 10 mg)*	OK	L3			*
Nature's Bounty Sleep[3] Tri-Layer Melatonin *(chamomile / lavender / lemon balm / L-theanine / melatonin - 10 mg / valerian)*	UNSAFE	L3			
Simply Sleep Nighttime Sleep Aid Caplets *(diphenhydramine)*	OK	L2	*		
Sleepinal Capsules *(diphenhydramine)*	OK	L2	*		
Sominex Maximum Strength Caplets / Original Formula Tablets *(diphenhydramine)*	OK	L2	*		

* *Additional note applies*   151   OK *OK to use*   UNSAFE *Do not use*

		SAFETY LEVEL (P. 19)	MONITOR INFANT FOR DROWS- INESS	LOOK FOR ALTERNATIVE THAT DOES NOT COMBINE INGREDIENTS	DO NOT EXCEED MELATONIN DOSE OF 3 mg PER DAY
Tylenol PM Extra Strength Caplets / PM Extra Strength Liquid *(acetaminophen / diphenhydramine)*	OK	L2	✳	✳	
Unisom SleepGels Softgels / SleepMelts Tablets *(diphenhydramine)*	OK	L2	✳		
Unisom SleepTabs Tablets *(doxylamine)*	OK	L3	✳		
Vicks ZzzQuil LiquiCaps / Nighttime Sleep Aid Liquid *(diphenhydramine)*	OK	L2	✳		
Vicks ZzzQuil Night Pain GelTabs / Night Pain Liquid *(acetaminophen / diphenhydramine)*	OK	L2	✳	✳	
Vicks ZzzQuil Pure Zzzs Melatonin Gummies / Pure Zzzs Melatonin Tablets *(chamomile / lavender / lemon balm / melatonin - 2 mg or 6 mg / valerian)*	OK	L3			✳
Vicks ZzzQuil Ultra Tablets *(doxylamine)*	OK	L3	✳		
Walgreens Headache Relief PM Tablets *(acetaminophen / diphenhydramine)*	OK	L2	✳	✳	
Zarbee's Naturals Sleep with Melatonin Gummies *(honey / melatonin - 3 mg)*	OK	L2			✳

Smoking Cessation Aids

Information Capsules:

 Nicotine replacement products, used as aids to help quit smoking, are usually compatible with breastfeeding. Negligible amounts of nicotine from smoking cessation aids appear in breastmilk. The amount of nicotine that transfers to breastmilk from these products is much less than the amount received from smoking cigarettes.

 None of the other toxic ingredients found in cigarettes are present in smoking cessation aids.

 For **ALL PRODUCTS** listed below, follow directions carefully and do not smoke during or in between use.

		SAFETY LEVEL (PAGE 19)
Habitrol Nicotine Transdermal System Patch Step 1 / Patch Step 2 / Patch Step 3 *(nicotine)*	OK	L3
NicoDerm CQ Step 1 Clear Patch / CQ Step 2 Clear Patch / CQ Step 3 Clear Patch *(nicotine)*	OK	L3
Nicorette 2 mg Gum / 4 mg Gum *(nicotine polacrilex)*	OK	L3
Nicorette 2 mg Lozenges / 4 mg Lozenges *(nicotine polacrilex)*	OK	L3
Nicorette 2 mg Patch / 4 mg Patch *(nicotine)*	OK	L3
Nicotine gum, generic *(nicotine polacrilex)*	OK	L3
Nicotine lozenges, generic *(nicotine polacrilex)*	OK	L3
Nicotine transdermal system patches, generic *(nicotine)*	OK	L3
Nicotrol Gum *(nicotine polacrilex)*	OK	L3

Stimulant Tablets

Information Capsules:

 It is fine to ingest caffeine while breastfeeding, however, **ALL PRODUCTS** listed below contain very high amounts. A caffeine dose of less than 150 mg, taken two or three times per day, has no apparent effect on a breastfeeding infant. Regular strength coffee, tea, or caffeinated soda is recommended in place of the products below.

 See page 195 for further safety information on caffeinated drinks.

	SAFETY LEVEL (PAGE 19)	
No Doz Tablets *(caffeine, 200 mg)*	UNSAFE	L2
Prolab Caffeine Tablets *(caffeine, 200 mg)*	UNSAFE	L2
Vivarin Tablets *(caffeine, 200 mg)*	UNSAFE	L2

Topical Analgesic (Pain Reliever) Balms

		SAFETY LEVEL (PAGE 19)	DO NOT APPLY TO BREASTS
Absorbine Jr. Pain Relief Back Patch / Pain Relieving Liquid / Ultra Strength Pain Relief Patch *(menthol / thymol)*	OK	L2	✱
ActivOn Ultra Strength Backache Roll-On Liquid *(camphor / menthol)*	OK	L2	✱
Arnicare Bruise Relief Cream / Pain Relief Cream / Pain Relief Gel *(Arnica montana)*	OK	L3	✱
ArthriCare Cream *(capsaicin)*	OK	L3	✱
Arthritis Hot Pain Relief Creme *(menthol / methylsalicylate)*	OK	L3	✱
Aspercreme Arthritis Pain Reliever Gel *(diclofenac sodium)*	OK	L2	✱
Aspercreme Original Pain Relief Cream *(trolamine salicylate)*	OK	L3	✱
Australian Dream Arthritis Pain Relief Cream *(aloe / chamomile / emu oil / ginger / turmeric)*	OK	L3	✱
BENGAY Greaseless Cream *(menthol / methylsalicylate)*	OK	L3	✱
BENGAY Ultra Strength Cream *(camphor / menthol / methylsalicylate)*	OK	L3	✱
Biofreeze Pain Relief Cream / Pain Relieving Gel / Pain Relieving Spray *(menthol)*	OK	L1	✱
Blue Emu Super Strength Original Cream *(aloe / emu oil / glucosamine / methylsufonylmethane)*	OK	L3	✱
Calendula cream, generic *(calendula)*	OK	L1	✱
Capzasin-HP Arthritis Pain Relief Crème *(capsaicin)*	OK	L3	✱
Icy Hot Original Large Patch / Original No Mess Pain Relief Roll On / Original Vanishing Scent Pain Relief Gel *(menthol)*	OK	L2	✱
Icy Hot Original Pain Relief Balm / Original Pain Relief Cream *(menthol / methylsalicylate)*	OK	L3	✱
JointFlex Pain Relief Cream *(camphor)*	OK	L2	✱
Mentholatum Pain Gel / Pain Patch *(methylsalicylate)*	OK	L3	✱
Mineral Ice Pain Relieving Gel *(menthol)*	OK	L2	✱
Myoflex Pain Relieving Cream *(trolamine salicylate)*	OK	L3	✱

✱ *Additional note applies*   155   OK *OK to use*   UNSAFE *Do not use*

		SAFETY LEVEL (PAGE 19)	DO NOT APPLY TO BREASTS
Salonpas Arthritis Pain Patch / Pain Relief Patch *(menthol / methylsalicylate)*	OK	L3	*
Sportscreme Cream *(trolamine salicylate)*	OK	L3	*
Thera-Gesic Cream *(menthol / methylsalicylate)*	OK	L3	*
Theraworx Relief for Muscle Cramps and Spasms *(magnesium sulfate)*	OK	L1	*
ThermaCare HeatWraps *(camphor / capsicum oleoresin)*	OK	L3	*
Tiger Balm Red Extra Strength Pain Relieving Ointment / Ultra Strength Pain Relieving Ointment *(cajuput oil / camphor / clove oil / menthol)*	OK	L2	*
Topricin Pain Relief Cream *(Arnica montana / homeopathic herbs)*	OK	L3	*
Traumeel Cream *(Arnica montana / homeopathic herbs)*	OK	L3	*
T-Relief Pain Relief Cream *(Arnica montana / homeopathic herbs / natural oils)*	OK	L3	*
Trixaicin HP Cream *(capsaicin)*	OK	L3	*
Unicity CM Plex Cream *(cetylated fatty acids / fish oil / soy)*	OK	L1	*
Voltaren Gel *(diclofenac sodium)*	OK	L2	*
Zostrix Arthritis Cream *(capsaicin)*	OK	L3	*

Topical Antifungals

Information Capsules:

 For **ALL PRODUCTS** listed below, if applied to the nipple or areola, clean the area with warm water and mild soap before breastfeeding.

		SAFETY LEVEL (PAGE 19)
Clotrimazole cream, generic *(clotrimazole)*	OK	L1
Desenex Antifungal Powder *(miconazole)*	OK	L2
Desenex Cream *(clotrimazole)*	OK	L1
FungiCure Anti-Fungal Liquid *(tolnaftate)*	OK	L2
FungiCure Anti-Fungal Liquid Gel / Intensive Anti-Fungal Treatment Spray *(clotrimazole)*	OK	L1
Fungi-Nail Anti-Fungal Liquid Solution / Anti-Fungal Ointment *(tolnaftate)*	OK	L2
Gordochom Solution *(chloroxylenol / undecylenic acid)*	OK	L2
Ketoconazole cream, generic *(ketoconazole)*	OK	L2
Lamisil AT Continuous Spray / Cream / Gel *(terbinafine)*	OK	L2
Lotrimin AF Antifungal Athlete's Foot Liquid Spray / Antifungal Athlete's Foot Powder / Antifungal Athlete's Foot Powder Spray / Antifungal Jock Itch Powder Spray *(miconazole)*	OK	L2
Lotrimin AF For Athlete's Foot Antifungal Cream / For Jock Itch Antifungal Cream / For Ringworm Antifungal Cream *(clotrimazole)*	OK	L1
Lotrimin Ultra Antifungal Athlete's Foot Cream / Ultra Antifungal Jock Itch Cream *(butenafine)*	OK	L2
Micatin Antifungal Cream *(miconazole)*	OK	L2
Miconazole cream, generic *(miconazole)*	OK	L2
Miracle of Aloe Miracure Anti-Fungal Liquid *(aloe / tolnaftate)*	OK	L2
Nizoral Topical Cream *(ketoconazole)*	OK	L2
Odor-Eaters Spray Powder *(tolnaftate)*	OK	L2

✳ *Additional note applies*

OK *OK to use* UNSAFE *Do not use*

		SAFETY LEVEL (PAGE 19)
Tinactin Antifungal Athlete's Foot Cream / Antifungal Athlete's Foot Deodorant Powder Spray / Antifungal Athlete's Foot Liquid Spray / Antifungal Athlete's Foot Powder Spray / Antifungal Jock Itch Cream / Antifungal Jock Itch Powder Spray *(tolnaftate)*	OK	L2
Tineacide Antifungal Cream *(miconazole)*	OK	L2
Zeasorb AF Antifungal Athlete's Foot Super Absorbent Powder / Antifungal Jock Itch Super Absorbent Powder *(miconazole)*	OK	L2

Topical Anti-Inflammatory and Anti-Itch Products

Information Capsules:

 For **ALL PRODUCTS** listed below that can be safely applied to breasts, if applied to the nipple or areola, clean the area with warm water and mild soap before breastfeeding.

		SAFETY LEVEL (PAGE 19)	DO NOT APPLY TO BREASTS
Aveeno 1% Hydrocortisone Anti-Itch Cream *(hydrocortisone)*	OK	L2	
Aveeno Anti-Itch Concentrated Lotion *(calamine / camphor / dimethicone / pramoxine)*	OK	L3	✳
Aveeno Eczema Therapy Daily Moisturizing Cream *(ceramides / colloidal oatmeal / dimethicone / glycerin / petrolatum)*	OK	L1	
Benadryl Extra Strength Itch Cooling Spray / Extra Strength Itch Relief Stick / Extra Strength Itch Stopping Cream / Original Strength Itch Stopping Cream *(diphenhydramine hydrochloride / zinc acetate)*	OK	L1	✳
Benadryl Extra Strength Itch Stopping Gel *(diphenhydramine hydrochloride)*	OK	L1	
Caladryl Clear Skin Protectant Lotion *(pramoxine / zinc acetate)*	OK	L2	✳
Caladryl Skin Protectant Lotion *(calamine / pramoxine)*	OK	L3	✳
Calamine lotion, generic *(calamine / zinc oxide)*	OK	L3	✳
CeraVe Eczema Relief Creamy Oil *(allantoin / colloidal oatmeal)*	OK	L1	
CeraVe Hydrocortisone Anti-Itch Cream *(hydrocortisone)*	OK	L2	
CeraVe Itch Relief Moisturizing Cream *(pramoxine / shea butter)*	OK	L2	✳
CeraVe Itch Relief Moisturizing Lotion *(allantoin / dimethicone / pramoxine)*	OK	L2	✳
Cetaphil Eczema Restoraderm Soothing Moisturizer *(allantoin / colloidal oatmeal / glycerin / shea butter / sunflower oil)*	OK	L1	
Cortizone-10 Maximum Strength Anti-Itch Liquid / Maximum Strength Cooling Relief Gel / Maximum Strength Intensive Healing Itch Relief Creme / Maximum Strength Itch Relief Ointment *(hydrocortisone)*	OK	L2	

		SAFETY LEVEL (PAGE 19)	DO NOT APPLY TO BREASTS
Cortizone-10 Maximum Strength Anti-Itch Lotion for Diabetics' Skin / Maximum Strength Anti-Itch Lotion for Psoriasis / Maximum Strength Intensive Healing Lotion for Eczema *(dimethicone / hydrocortisone)*	OK	L2	
Dermarest Eczema Medicated Lotion *(hydrocortisone)*	OK	L2	
Domeboro Rash Relief Medicated Soak Powder Packets *(aluminum sulfate / calcium acetate)*	OK	L2	✱
Dr. Nice's Moisturizing Gel *(peppermint oil / poloxamer 407)*	OK	L1	
Eucerin Eczema Relief Body Cream *(castor oil / Glycyrrhiza inflata root extract / piroctone olamine)*	OK	L2	✱
Eucerin Itch Relief Intensive Calming Lotion *(dimethicone / menthol)*	OK	L1	✱
Eucerin Skin Calming Itch Relief Treatment Lotion *(colloidal oatmeal / dimethicone)*	OK	L1	
Gold Bond Medicated Anti-Itch Body Lotion / Medicated Rapid Relief Anti-Itch Cream *(menthol / pramoxine)*	OK	L2	✱
Gold Bond Medicated Body Lotion / Medicated Extra Strength Body Lotion *(dimethicone / menthol)*	OK	L1	✱
Gold Bond Medicated Eczema Relief Skin Protectant Cream *(aloe / colloidal oatmeal / dimethicone / ginger / glycerin / petrolatum / shea butter)*	OK	L1	
Gold Bond Medicated Extra Strength Body Powder / Medicated Original Strength Body Powder *(menthol / zinc oxide)*	OK	L2	✱
Gold Bond Medicated Maximum Strength Pain & Itch Relief Cream *(lidocaine)*	OK	L2	✱
Hydrocortisone cream 0.5% / hydrocortisone cream 1%, generic *(hydrocortisone)*	OK	L2	
Hydrocortisone lotion 0.5% / hydrocortisone lotion 1%, generic *(hydrocortisone)*	OK	L2	
Hydrocortisone ointment 0.5% / hydrocortisone ointment 1%, generic *(hydrocortisone)*	OK	L2	
Ivarest Poison Ivy Itch Cream Double Relief Formula *(benzyl alcohol / calamine / diphenhydramine)*	OK	L3	✱
Ivy-Dry Anti-Itch Cream with Zytrel / Cream with Zytrel *(camphor / menthol / zinc acetate)*	OK	L2	✱
Ivy-Dry Cream / Super *(benzyl alcohol / camphor / cetyl alcohol / menthol / propylene glycol)*	OK	L2	✱

		SAFETY LEVEL (PAGE 19)	DO NOT APPLY TO BREASTS
Ivy-Dry Soap *(aloe / colloidal oatmeal / sodium tallowate)*	OK	L2	
Ivy-Dry Super Continuous Spray *(benzyl alcohol / camphor / zinc acetate)*	OK	L2	✳
IvyX Pre-Contact Skin Solution *(aloe / propylene glycol)*	OK	L2	✳
Lanacane Medicated Cream *(benzocaine)*	OK	L1	✳
MG217 Eczema Body Cream *(allantoin / colloidal oatmeal / shea butter)*	OK	L1	
Sarna Eczema Relief Anti-Itch Whipped Foam *(hydrocortisone)*	OK	L2	
Sarna Original Itch Relief Moisturizing Lotion *(camphor / menthol)*	OK	L2	✳
Sarna Sensitive Itch Relief Moisturizing Lotion *(pramoxine)*	OK	L2	✳
Sarna Sensitive Lotion *(pramoxine)*	OK	L2	✳
Scalpicin Maximum Strength Anti-Itch Liquid *(hydrocortisone / salicylic acid)*	OK	L3	✳
Tecnu Calagel Anti-Itch Gel *(benzethonium chloride / diphenhydramine hydrochloride / zinc acetate)*	OK	L2	✳
Tecnu Extreme Poison Ivy & Oak Scrub *(silicon dioxide)*	OK	L1	✳
Zanfel Poison Ivy, Oak & Sumac Wash *(nonoxynol-9 / polyethylene granules / sodium lauroyl sarcoosinate)*	OK	L3	✳
Zinc oxide ointment, generic *(zinc oxide)*	OK	L2	✳

Topical Antiseptics and Burn and Wound Care Products

Information Capsules:

For **ALL PRODUCTS** listed below that can be safely applied to breasts, if applied to the nipple or areola, clean the area with warm water and mild soap before breastfeeding.

		SAFETY LEVEL (PAGE 19)	DO NOT APPLY TO BREASTS	AVOID BREATHING FUMES
Alocane Maximum Strength Emergency Burn Gel *(lidocaine)*	OK	L2	∗	
A+D Original Ointment *(lanolin / petrolatum / vitamin A / vitamin D)*	OK	L1		
Aquaphor Healing Ointment *(ceresin / glycerin / lanolin / mineral oil / petrolatum)*	OK	L2		
Bacitracin ointment, generic *(bacitracin)*	OK	L1		
Bacitraycin Plus Maximum Strength Pain Relief *(aloe / bacitracin / petrolatum / pramoxine)*	OK	L2	∗	
Bacitraycin Plus Ointment *(aloe / bacitracin / mineral oil / petrolatum)*	OK	L1		
Bactine Max Pain Relieving Cleansing Liquid / Max Pain Relieving Cleansing Spray *(benzalkonium chloride / lidocaine)*	OK	L3	∗	
BAND-AID First Aid Antiseptic To-Go-Spray *(benzalkonium chloride / pramoxine)*	OK	L3	∗	
Betadine Antiseptic Cream / Antiseptic Dry Powder Spray / Antiseptic Solution / Antiseptic Spray *(povidone iodine)*	OK	L1		
Boil Ease Ointment *(benzocaine / camphor / eucalyptus / menthol / petrolatum / thymol)*	OK	L2	∗	
Burn Jel Max Emergency Burn Care Pain Relieving Gel *(aloe / lidocaine)*	OK	L2	∗	

		SAFETY LEVEL (PAGE 19)	DO NOT APPLY TO BREASTS	AVOID BREATHING FUMES
Calamine lotion, generic *(calamine / zinc oxide)*	OK	L3	*	
Campho-Phenique Pain and Itch Relief Antiseptic Gel / Pain and Itch Relief Antiseptic Liquid *(camphorated phenol)*	UNSAFE	L4		
Clorpactin WCS-90 Solution *(sodium oxychlorosene)*	OK	L3	*	
Curad FlexSEAL Spray Bandage *(ethyl alcohol / methane oxybis)*	OK	L3	*	*
Dermoplast Hospital Strength First Aid Antibacterial Spray *(aloe / benzethonium chloride / benzocaine)*	OK	L1	*	
Dermoplast Hospital Strength Pain, Burn & Itch Spray / Insect Itch & Sting Relief Spray / Sunburn & Burn Relief Spray *(aloe / benzocaine / lanolin / menthol)*	OK	L1	*	
Dr. Nice's Moisturizing Gel *(peppermint oil / poloxamer 407)*	OK	L1		
Epsal Drawing Salve Ointment *(alcohol / lanolin / magnesium sulfate / mineral oil / white petrolatum)*	OK	L1		
Foille Medicated First Aid Ointment *(benzocaine / chloroxylenol)*	OK	L3	*	
Hibiclens Antiseptic Skin Cleanser Liquid *(chlorhexidine gluconate / isopropyl alcohol)*	UNSAFE	L4		
Hydrogen peroxide topical solution, generic *(hydrogen peroxide)*	OK	L1		
Hyland's Naturals Pain Relief and Irritant Drawing Salve *(ethyl alcohol / homeopathic herbs)*	OK	L2	*	
Lidocaine cream, generic *(lidocaine)*	OK	L2	*	
NeilMed Neilcleanse Wound Wash *(sodium chloride)*	OK	L1		
NEOSPORIN Original Ointment *(bacitracin / neomycin / polymyxin B)*	OK	L2		
NEOSPORIN + Burn Relief Ointment / + Pain Relief Ointment *(bacitracin / neomycin / polymyxin B / pramoxine)*	OK	L2	*	
NEOSPORIN + Pain Relief Cream *(neomycin / polymyxin B / pramoxine)*	OK	L2	*	

* *Additional note applies*   163   OK *OK to use*   UNSAFE *Do not use*

		SAFETY LEVEL (PAGE 19)	DO NOT APPLY TO BREASTS	AVOID BREATHING FUMES
New-Skin Liquid Bandage *(8-hydroxyquinolone)*	OK	L2	✻	✻
New-Skin Liquid Bandage Spray *(benzethonium chloride)*	OK	L1	✻	
Nexcare No Sting Liquid Bandage *(acrylate terpolymer / hexamethyldisiloxane / polyphenylmethylsiloxane)*	OK	L3	✻	✻
Petroleum jelly, generic *(white petrolatum)*	OK	L1		
POLYSPORIN First Aid Antibiotic Ointment *(bacitracin / polymyxin B)*	OK	L2		
Povidone iodine ointment / solution, generic *(povidone iodine)*	OK	L1	✻	
Prosacea Rosacea Treatment Gel *(aloe / sulfur / urea)*	OK	L2	✻	
Triple antibiotic ointment, generic *(bacitracin / neomycin / polymyxin B)*	OK	L2		
Vaseline Original Healing Jelly *(white petrolatum)*	OK	L1		

Vaginal Health Products

		SAFETY LEVEL (PAGE 19)
Astroglide Gel *(chlorhexidine / glycerin / hydroxymethylcellulose)*	OK	L3
AZO Yeast Plus Tablets *(homeopathic herbs)*	OK	L3
Clotrimazole 3 vaginal cream, generic *(clotrimazole)*	OK	L1
Clotrimazole 7 vaginal cream, generic *(clotrimazole)*	OK	L1
Cortizone-10 Feminine Itch Relief Cream *(hydrocortisone)*	OK	L2
Damiva Vaginal Suppository *(calendula / cocoa butter / hamamelis / sugar)*	OK	L2
Florajen Acidophilus Probiotic Supplement *(lactobacillus)*	OK	L1
Florajen Digestion Probiotic Supplement *(bifidobacterium lactis / bifidobacterium longum / lactobacillus)*	OK	L1
Florajen Women Probiotic Supplement *(lactobacillus)*	OK	L1
Jarro-Dophilus Women Probiotic Supplement *(lactobacillus)*	OK	L1
K-Y Jelly Classic Water-Based Personal Lubricant *(hydroxycellulose)*	OK	L1
Lubrigyn Cream *(calendula / cocamidopropyl betaine / dimethicone / imidazolidinyl urea / lactic acid / sweet almond oil / propylene glycol)*	OK	L3
Luvena Vaginal Moisturizer & Lubricant *(cranberry / d-mannose / glycogen / jojoba oil / lactic acid / lactoferrin / vitamin E)*	OK	L3
Miconazole 7 vaginal cream, generic *(miconazole)*	OK	L2
MONISTAT 1 Combination Pack Ovule *(miconazole)*	OK	L2
MONISTAT 1 Tioconazole Ointment *(tioconazole)*	OK	L2
MONISTAT 3 Combination Pack Ovule / Combination Pack Prefilled Cream / Combination Pack Suppository / Prefilled Cream *(miconazole)*	OK	L2
MONISTAT 7 Combination Pack Cream / Prefilled Cream *(miconazole)*	OK	L2
MONISTAT Care Instant Itch Relief Cream *(hydrocortisone)*	OK	L2
RepHresh Pro-B Probiotic *(lactobacillus acidophilus)*	OK	L1
Replens Long-Lasting Vaginal Moisturizer *(polycarbophil)*	OK	L1
Summer's Eve Daily Cleansing Wash / Daily Gentle Wash / Daily Refreshing Wash / Daily Wash *(preservatives and/or scents / water)*	OK	L1
Summer's Eve Daily Gentle Cloths / Daily Individual Cloths / Daily Refreshing Cloths *(preservatives and/or scents / water)*	OK	L1

✱ *Additional note applies*   165   OK *OK to use*   UNSAFE *Do not use*

		SAFETY LEVEL (PAGE 19)
Summer's Eve Extra Cleansing Vinegar and Water Douche *(vinegar / water)*	OK	L2
Taro 7 Day Vaginal Cream *(clotrimazole)*	OK	L1
Taro Miconazole Nitrate 2% Vaginal Cream *(miconazole)*	OK	L2
Tioconazole 1 vaginal ointment, generic *(tioconazole)*	OK	L2
Vagisil All-Day Fresh Wash / Daily Intimate Wash / Healthy Detox All Over Wash *(mild detergents)*	OK	L2
Vagisil Anti-Itch Medicated Wipes *(pramoxine)*	OK	L2
Vagisil Hydrocortisone Anti-Itch Creme for Sensitive Skin *(hydrocortisone)*	OK	L2
Vagisil Long Lasting Moisturizing Lubricant *(glycerin)*	OK	L2
Vagisil Maximum Strength Anti-Itch Creme / Regular Strength Moisturizing Anti-Itch Creme *(benzocaine / resorcinol)*	OK	L2
Vagistat 1 Dose Treatment Vaginal Ointment *(tioconazole)*	OK	L2
Vagistat 3 Day Treatment Combination Pack / 7 Day Treatment Vaginal Cream *(miconazole)*	OK	L2
YeastGard Douche *(homeopathic herbs)*	OK	L1
YeastGard Gel Treatment / Suppositories *(homeopathic herbs)*	OK	L1
YeastGard Homeopathic Medicine Capsules *(homeopathic herbs)*	OK	L1

6.

HERBAL REMEDIES AND PRODUCTS

Natural Does Not Mean Safe

Like prescription drugs and OTC medications, consumers use herbal remedies and products to treat a variety of ailments and maintain their health. The use of herbals is as prevalent among breastfeeding parents as any other consumers. Herbals are readily available and provide alternatives to prescription or OTC medications.

That being said, nursing families should approach the use of herbals with caution. The fact that many manufacturers promote their products as "natural" does not necessarily imply that using them is safe or compatible with breastfeeding.

The Food and Drug Administration (FDA) does not regulate herbal products in the same manner as prescription and OTC medicines. Instead, the FDA regulates herbals under food manufacturing regulations. Herbal products are required to be free of contaminants, and herbal labels are not allowed to make unfounded health and medical claims, but there is no government regulation of herbals as drugs.

Because of this, active ingredients may be present in greater or lesser amounts than the herbal package label lists. Unknown harmful ingredients may also be present. Strengths of herbal product ingredients may vary depending upon the particular plant used; the part of the plant used; and where, when, and how the herb was processed. These inconsistencies can lead to differences in efficacy and potentially harmful effects in breastfeeding parents and/or their infants.

In reality, most knowledge about potential side effects of the wide variety of herbals comes from a systematic collection of data in Germany (e.g., *The Complete German Commission E Monographs: Therapeutic Guide to Herbal Medicines*, which has been translated into English). There have been reports of specific adverse effects that are caused by herbals, but there is still no standard way to report these adverse effects. Information provided on the use of herbals should serve as general guidelines for nursing mothers.

In addition to the many everyday health uses of herbal products, lactation consultants often recommend (and breastfeeding mothers often use) herbals called galactagogues to help increase milk supply. Commonly used galactagogues include blessed thistle, chaste tree fruit, fennel, fenugreek, garlic, rue, and milk thistle. Other herbals that may act as galactagogues include alfalfa, anise, borage, caraway, coriander, dandelion, dill, fennel, hops, marshmallow root, nettle, oat straw, red clover, red raspberry, and vervain.

As with all medications, breastfeeding parents should have a real need for treatment before taking herbal preparations. Depending on the condition being treated, conventional medications should be considered first-line therapy until more controlled studies and data are available for specific herbals.

CAUTION! Like any other drug, all herbal preparations may:

- Interact negatively with other prescription or nonprescription drugs

- Affect or worsen certain health conditions

- Cause allergic reactions

- Reduce milk production

It is especially important to talk to your healthcare provider before using herbal products if you are taking any medications or have any known health conditions or allergies.

Herbal Galactagogues
(Used to Increase Milk Supply)

Note: Many factors can affect milk supply and maintenance. It is not unheard of for a galactagogue to have no effect or to even decrease milk supply, depending on the individual. If a galactagogue you are taking is not working for you, switch to another galactagogue or combine with additional galactagogues. Talk to a lactation consultant about additional strategies to increase milk supply.

OK Alfalfa (*Medicago sativa*)

USE: Galactagogue, diuretic, laxative

DOSE: Up to 60 g daily (1 to 2 capsules taken 4 times daily)

CAUTION: *Monitor infant for potential side effects.* Alfalfa may cause loose stools and/or photosensitivity; do not use if allergic to peanuts and/or legumes; do not use if affected by systemic lupus erythematosus (SLE).

OK Anise Seed (*Pimpinella anisum*)

USE: Galactagogue, anxiety relief, antiflatulent

DOSE: 3.5 g to 7 g taken 5 to 6 times a day, infused in tincture or tea

CAUTION: *Monitor infant for potential side effects*. Anise may cause allergic reaction.

OK Ashwagandha (*Withania somnifera*)

USE: Galactagogue, anti-inflammatory, sedative

DOSE: 3 g to 6 g daily of dried root/powder boiled in 2 cups of water until reduced to 1 cup

CAUTION: May interact with some drugs. Use caution with gastrointestinal disorders.

OK Barley (*Hordeum vulgare*)

USE: Galactagogue (specifically aids in milk let down), anxiety relief, sleep aid

DOSE: 15 g daily of barley extract, or 1 cup to 2 cups daily of tea, or 1 daily bottle of beer

CAUTION: Do not use fermented barley if suffering from depression.

OK Blessed Thistle (*Cnicus benedictus*)

USE: Galactagogue, may increase appetite and settle upset stomach

DOSE: Up to 2 g daily, in capsule form

CAUTION: *Monitor infant for potential side effects.* Blessed thistle may cause allergic reaction.

OK Borage (*Borago officinalis*)

USE: Galactagogue, anxiety relief, diuretic

DOSE: 1 g to 2 g daily, in capsule form or infused in tincture

CAUTION: *Monitor infant for potential side effects.* Borage may cause loose stools and/or minor gastrointestinal upset; avoid large amounts due to potential blood thinner action.

OK Brewer's Yeast (*Saccharomyces cerevisiae*)

USE: Galactagogue, antidiarrheal, for treatment of acne

DOSE: 250 mg to 750 mg daily, added to food or drinks

CAUTION: Brewer's yeast may cause allergic reaction; may cause flatulence.

OK Caraway Seed (*Carum carvi*)

USE: Galactagogue, anxiety relief, antiflatulent

DOSE: 1.5 g to 6 g daily, infused in tincture, tea, or essential oil

CAUTION: Avoid large amounts of the essential oil form.

OK Chasteberry / Vitex (*Vitex agnus-castus*)

USE: Galactagogue, for treatment of breast pain, for dysmenorrhea

DOSE: 30 mg to 40 mg daily as an alcoholic extract (50% to 70% alcohol)

CAUTION: *Monitor infant for potential side effects.* Herb may cause rash; extract form has high alcohol content, although amount consumed is very small.

OK Clove (*Syzygium aromaticum*)

USE: Galactagogue, topical anesthetic, for treatment of oral mucosa inflammation

DOSE: For galactagogue effect, use ground cloves occasionally as spice in food / Topically, dilute no more than 6 drops of clove oil in 1 oz of carrier oil or cream

CAUTION: None when used as a spice; do not use oil repeatedly or in large amounts.

OK Coriander / Cilantro Seed (*Coriandrum sativum*)

USE: Galactagogue, antiflatulent, diuretic, mild antidiabetic

DOSE: 3 g daily, infused in tea

CAUTION: *Monitor infant for potential side effects.* Herb may (rarely) cause photosensitivity; avoid herb if allergic to celery; avoid large amounts of herb.

OK Dandelion (*Taraxacum officinale*)

USE: Galactagogue, antidiabetic, diuretic

DOSE: 5 g taken 3 times daily, in capsule form or infused in tincture or tea

CAUTION: *Monitor infant for potential side effects.* Dandelion may rarely cause contact dermatitis; do not use if affected by bile duct blockage, gall bladder problems, or bowel obstruction.

OK Dill Seed (*Anethum graveolens*)

USE: Galactagogue (specifically aids in milk ejection), antiflatulent, diuretic

DOSE: 3 g daily infused in tincture or tea

CAUTION: None known

OK Fennel Seed (*Foeniculum vulgare*)

USE: Galactagogue, for gastrointestinal disorders, expectorant

DOSE: 0.1 mL to 0.6 mL (equal to 100 mg to 600 mg) daily as oil

CAUTION: *Monitor infant for potential side effects.* Fennel may cause allergic reaction and dermatitis.

OK Fenugreek Seed (*Trigonella foenum-graecum*)

USE: Galactagogue, may stimulate appetite, topical anti-inflammatory

DOSE: Orally, 6 g daily in capsule form / Topically, 50 g mixed with 8 oz of water

CAUTION: *Monitor infant for potential side effects.* Do not use if allergic to peanuts and/or legumes; fenugreek may cause nausea and vomiting in parent and diarrhea in breastfed baby; may increase asthma symptoms or lower glucose levels in parent; may cause skin reactions with external use (avoid nipple area); may cause "maple syrup" smell in parent's and/or baby's urine and/or sweat. Monitor parent if diagnosed with a thyroid disorder.

`OK` Flaxseed / Linseed (*Linum usitatissimum*)

USE: Galactagogue, for chronic constipation, for gastritis, topical anti-inflammatory

DOSE: Orally, 5 g to 50 g daily as whole or ground seeds, or 2.5 g daily as oil / Topically, 30 g to 50 g as a paste

CAUTION: Flaxseed may cause allergic reaction.

`OK` Garlic Bulb (*Allium sativum*)

USE: Galactagogue, possible positive cardiovascular effects and/or immune system stimulation

DOSE: 4 g to 9 g daily in capsule form

CAUTION: Garlic may decrease nursing time due to odor in breastmilk.

`OK` Goat's Rue (*Galega officinalis*)

USE: Galactagogue, for lowering blood glucose levels

DOSE: 1 mL to 2 mL of tincture taken 2 to 3 times daily

CAUTION: None known

`OK` Hops (*Humulus lupulus*)

USE: Galactagogue (specifically aids in milk let down), anxiety relief, sleep aid

DOSE: 500 mg daily of dry extract, or 1 cup to 2 cups daily of tea, or 1 daily bottle of beer

CAUTION: *Monitor infant for potential side effects.* Do not use fermented hops if suffering from depression.

`OK` Marshmallow Root (*Althea officinalis*)

USE: Galactagogue, diuretic

DOSE: Two 500 mg capsules taken 3 times daily, or 60 g daily infused in tincture or tea

CAUTION: *Monitor infant for potential side effects.* Marshmallow root may (rarely) cause allergic reaction.

`OK` Milk Thistle (*Silybum marianum*)

USE: Galactagogue, possible liver protective properties

DOSE: 12 g to 15 g daily in infusion (equal to 200 mg to 400 mg of silibinin)

CAUTION: *Monitor infant for potential side effects.* Milk thistle may have laxative effect and/or cause allergic reaction.

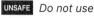

OK **Moghat (*Glossostemon bruguieri*)**

USE: Galactagogue, antimicrobial, diuretic, for gout

DOSE: 50 g (3 tbsp) daily of powder in traditional hot drink

CAUTION: None known

OK **Moringa / Malunggay (*Moringa oleifera*)**

USE: Galactagogue, antidiabetic, analgesic, antioxidant

DOSE: 250 mg taken 2 times daily, in capsule form or infused in tea

CAUTION: Do not mega-dose to avoid potential drug interactions.

OK **Oat Straw / Oat Tops (*Avena sativa*)**

USE: Galactagogue, diuretic, anxiety relief, antidepressant

DOSE: 100 g daily infused in tea or tincture

CAUTION: Should not be used by those with celiac disease.

OK **Quinoa (*Chenopodium quinoa*)**

USE: Galactagogue, urinary tract disinfectant

DOSE: 45 g daily as cooked seeds, flour in baked goods, or powder in drinks

CAUTION: None known

OK **Red Clover (*Trifolium pratense*)**

USE: Galactagogue, for estrogenic properties, expectorant

DOSE: 40 mg to 80 mg daily infused in tincture or tea

CAUTION: Do not exceed recommended dosage; avoid fermented red clover; do not use if taking anticoagulants and/or aspirin (contains coumarin, a blood thinner).

OK **Red Raspberry Leaf (*Rubus idaeus*)**

USE: Galactagogue (may increase milk ejection), nutritive

DOSE: 2.7 g daily infused in tincture or tea, or three 300 mg capsules taken 3 times daily

CAUTION: *Monitor infant for potential side effects.* Red raspberry may (rarely) cause loose stools and/or nausea; may decrease milk supply if used for longer than 2 weeks.

 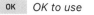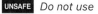

`OK` Sesame (*Sesamum indicum*)

USE: Galactagogue, digestive aid, for high blood pressure

DOSE: 9 g daily as seeds, or 35 g daily as oil

CAUTION: Sesame seeds and oil may cause allergic reaction.

`OK` Stinging Nettle (*Urtica dioica*) and Dwarf Nettle (*Urtica urens*)

USE: Galactagogue, mild diuretic, for mild gastrointestinal upset

DOSE: 1.8 g in the form of one 600 mg capsule taken 3 times daily, 2 cups to 3 cups of tea daily, or 2.5 mL to 5 mL of tincture taken 3 times daily

CAUTION: *Monitor infant for potential side effects.* Nettles may cause mild diuresis and/or mild gastrointestinal upset.

`OK` Turmeric (*Curcuma longa*)

USE: Galactagogue, for gastrointestinal upset

DOSE: 1.5 g to 2 g daily as a spice in food or drinks

CAUTION: May cause stomach upset, nausea, dizziness, or diarrhea, especially at higher doses.

`OK` Vervain (*Verbena officinalis*)

USE: Galactagogue, anxiety relief, for hypertension

DOSE: 30 g to 50 g daily infused in tea

CAUTION: None known

Other Commonly Used Herbal Remedies and Products

UNSAFE Alder Buckthorn Bark (*Rhamnus frangula*)

USE: Laxative

CAUTION: *Do not use if breastfeeding.* May cause gastrointestinal distress (short term use) and/or electrolyte imbalance, albuminuria, hematuria, potassium deficiency and/or irregular heartbeats.

UNSAFE Aloes (*Aloe barbadensis*, *Aloe ferox*, *Aloe perry*i, and *Aloe vera*)

USE: Laxative

CAUTION: *Do not ingest any form of aloe (latex or gel) if breastfeeding.* Aloes may cause gastrointestinal distress (short term use) and/or electrolyte imbalance, albuminuria, hematuria, potassium deficiency and/or irregular heartbeats.

NOTE: Topical gel (Aloe vera) may be safely used for sunburn, minor burns, bug bites, and to soften the skin.

UNSAFE Angelica Root / Dong Quai (*Angelica archangelica*)

USE: For stimulating the central nervous system, for regulating menstrual cycle (due to antispasmodic and vasodilatation effects)

CAUTION: *Do not use if breastfeeding.* Possible phytoestrogenic effect on infant (may interfere with hormones); herb can sensitize skin to light and UV radiation.

UNSAFE Bilberry (*Vaccinium myrtillus*)

USE: For eye health

CAUTION: *Do not use if breastfeeding.* Herb inhibits lactation. Do not use if taking blood thinners.

UNSAFE Black Walnut (*Juglans nigra*)

USE: Anti-infective, anti-inflammatory, for heart health

CAUTION: *Do not use if breastfeeding.* Black walnut inhibits lactation. May cause allergic reaction.

 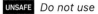

`OK` Bugleweed (*Lycopus americanus*)

USE: For breast pain and/or mild thyroid hyperfunction

STANDARD DOSE: 1 g to 2 g daily infused in tea, or 10 mg to 20 mg daily as extract

CAUTION: *Monitor infant for potential side effects. Herb may decrease prolactin levels, which may affect milk production.* Monitor mother and baby for thyroid enlargement after extended exposure.

`UNSAFE` Butterbur / Petasites Root (*Petasites hybridus*)

USE: For reducing migraine frequency, for treatment of acute spastic urinary tract pain and urinary tract stone pain

CAUTION: *Do not use if breastfeeding.* Herb is contraindicated due to potential liver toxicity.

`UNSAFE` Cascara Sagrada Bark (*Frangula purshiana*)

USE: Laxative

CAUTION: *Do not use if breastfeeding.* May cause gastrointestinal distress (short term use) and/or electrolyte imbalance, albuminuria, hematuria, potassium deficiency, and/or irregular heartbeats.

`OK` Chamomile Flower (*Matricaria chamomilla*)

USE: Calmative, for indigestion, for relaxation, topical anti-inflammatory

STANDARD DOSE: Orally, 3 g to 5 g infused in tea, taken 3 to 4 times daily / Topically, 50 g in 1.5 gallons of water as a bath additive, poultice, or rinse

CAUTION: None known

`UNSAFE` Coltsfoot Leaf (*Tussilago farfara*)

USE: Anti-inflammatory during respiratory disturbances

CAUTION: *Do not use if breastfeeding.* Possible liver toxicity. If taken when not breastfeeding, do not use for more than 4 to 6 weeks total per year.

`UNSAFE` Comfrey Leaf and Root (*Symphytum officinale*)

USE: Topical anti-inflammatory for bruised areas, sprains, and pulled muscles

CAUTION: *Do not use if breastfeeding.* Avoid due to liver toxicity and anti-mitotic effect (inhibits cell reproduction properties); do not use on sore nipples, breasts, or perineum.

 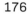

OK Cranberry (*Vaccinium macrocarpon*)

USE: Antibacterial and antiseptic to protect against and to resolve urinary tract infections

STANDARD DOSE: 100 mg to 500 mg taken 3 times a day, in capsule form or infused in tea

CAUTION: May cause allergic reaction. Avoid if taking blood thinners. Consuming large amounts of cranberry may cause digestive upset or kidney stones.

OK Echinacea Pallida Root (*Echinacea pallida*) and Echinacea Purpurea (*Echinacea purpurea*)

USE: For prevention of common cold, for wound healing, for treatment of uncomplicated lower urinary tract infections

STANDARD DOSE: 900 mg daily in capsule or tablet form, in juice, or infused in tea

CAUTION: Usually safe for breastfeeding if used for less than 8 weeks (if used for more than 8 weeks, echinacea may weaken immune-stimulating effects); those affected by tuberculosis, HIV, or autoimmune diseases should not use; avoid if allergic to sunflower.

OK Elderflower (*Sambucus nigra*)

USE: For acute upper respiratory infections, diaphoretic (increases sweating), expectorant

STANDARD DOSE: 10 g to 15 g daily infused in 1 cup to 2 cups of tea, 1.5 g to 3 g daily as fluid extract, or 2.5 g to 7.5 g daily infused in tincture

CAUTION: Elderflower appears to be safe for breastfeeding as long as only the flowers are used; in sufficient quantities, the seeds are toxic.

UNSAFE Ephedra (*Ephedra sinica*)

USE: Vitalizing and stimulating effects, for treatment of asthma and bronchoconstriction, for weight loss

CAUTION: *Do not use if breastfeeding.* Ephedra can cause vasoconstriction, rapid heart rate, and insomnia; a rapid decrease in effectiveness is possible; addiction is possible; no dose is considered safe, even while not breastfeeding.

NOTE: FDA ban and court actions have removed ephedra from the market, but illegal or foreign sources may still be available.

OK Evening Primrose Oil (*Oenothera biennis*)

USE: Anti-inflammatory, for relieving skin conditions, for PMS symptoms

STANDARD DOSE: 3 g to 8 g daily in divided doses, in capsule form (clinical effect may take 8 weeks to 12 weeks)

CAUTION: Hypersensitivity is possible; generally safe when used appropriately.

UNSAFE Feverfew (*Tanacetum parthenium*)

USE: For migraine headaches

CAUTION: *Do not use if breastfeeding.* Safety cannot be assured; mouth sores may occur; taste alterations and lip and tongue swelling/irritation are possible.

UNSAFE Flannel Weed (*Sida cordifolia*)

USE: Anti-inflammatory during respiratory disturbances

CAUTION: *Do not use if breastfeeding.* Herb inhibits lactation.

OK Flaxseed (Cracked or Ground) (*Linum usitatissimum*)

USE: Laxative

STANDARD DOSE: 1 tbsp daily mixed with 5 oz of water, or added to foods (may take several days for laxative effects)

NOTE: Flaxseed oil is a rich source of omega-3 fatty acids, which can prevent skin dryness when applied topically.

OK Ginger (*Zingiber officinale*)

USE: For motion sickness, for nausea and vomiting, for upset stomach

STANDARD DOSE: Two 500 mg capsules every 4 hours as needed

CAUTION: None known

OK Ginkgo Leaf (*Ginkgo biloba*)

USE: For memory and concentration, may enhance learning ability in younger people, may relieve altitude sickness with short-term (2 to 3 days) pretreatment

STANDARD DOSE: 120 mg daily in 2 or 3 divided doses, in capsule form

CAUTION: *Monitor infant for potential side effects.* Potential platelet inhibition, avoid for infants with cardiovascular disease and/or mothers already taking a blood thinner; do not use more than 6 to 8 weeks to determine if any benefit exists.

UNSAFE Ginseng Root (*Panax ginseng*)

USE: For enhancing mental ability

CAUTION: *Do not use if breastfeeding.* Ginseng may increase blood pressure in breastfeeding parent who already has hypertension; herb should not be used when breastfeeding due to estrogenic side effects from ginsenoside components.

OK Goldenrod (*Solidago canadensis*, *Solidago virgaurea*, *Solidago gigantea*)

USE: For treatment of lower urinary tract infections

STANDARD DOSE: 6 g to 12 g daily as botanical preparation or infused in tea

CAUTION: If used when breastfeeding, drink large amounts of water and/or fluids.

OK Grape Seed Extract (*Vitis vinifera*)

USE: Antioxidant, anti-inflammatory

STANDARD DOSE: Preventative, 50 mg daily in capsule form / Therapeutic, 150 mg to 300 mg daily in capsule form

CAUTION: Hypersensitivity to herb is possible; generally considered to be safe during breastfeeding when used appropriately.

OK Grapefruit Seed Extract (*Citrus x paradisi*)

USE: For treatment of thrush

STANDARD DOSE: 250 mg taken 3 times a day in capsule form or as liquid extract diluted in water (diluted liquid extract may also be applied topically to nipples after breastfeeding)

CAUTION: Hypersensitivity to herb is possible; generally considered to be safe during breastfeeding when used appropriately. Extract has bitter taste.

UNSAFE Hawthorn (*Crataegus laevigata*, *Crataegus monogyna*, *Crataegus oxyacantha*)

USE: For hypertension, for high cholesterol

CAUTION: *Do not use if breastfeeding.* No information available for breastfeeding; caution is advised.

 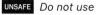

`UNSAFE` Holy Basil (*Ocimum tenuiflorum*)

USE: Anti-inflammatory, anxiety relief, antidiabetic

CAUTION: *Do not use if breastfeeding.* Herb inhibits lactation. Do not confuse with basil (*Cocimum basilicum*) that is commonly used in cooking.

`UNSAFE` Indian Snakeroot (*Rauvolfia serpentina*)

USE: Anxiety relief, tension relief, for treatment of psychomotor irritation and mild, essential hypertension

CAUTION: *Do not use if breastfeeding.* Possible central nervous system depression; may cause severe depression due to breakdown of norepinephrine.

`UNSAFE` Kava Kava Root (*Piper methysticum*)

USE: Anxiety relief, for restlessness

CAUTION: *Do not use if breastfeeding.* Possible central nervous system depression and/or liver damage; allergic reaction possible; possible sedation with large doses; long-term use of large doses may cause temporary discoloration of skin/hair/nails.

`OK` Lemon Balm (*Melissa officinalis*)

USE: Calmative, mild galactagogue, sleep aid

STANDARD DOSE: 1.5 g to 4.5 g infused in 5 oz of tea, taken up to to 4 times daily, especially at bedtime

CAUTION: None known

`UNSAFE` Licorice Root (*Glycyrrhiza glabra*)

USE: For treatment of peptic and duodenal ulcers

CAUTION: *Do not use if breastfeeding.* May cause sodium and water retention; may cause low potassium levels; may cause hypertension

NOTE: These precautions do not apply to eating licorice candy on occasion, following recommended serving sizes.

`UNSAFE` Osha Root (*Ligusticum porteri*)

USE: For treatment of respiratory infections

CAUTION: *Do not use if breastfeeding.* Herb inhibits lactation.

UNSAFE Parsley (*Petroselinum crispum*)

USE: For treatment of urinary tract infections, for improved digestion

CAUTION: *Do not use if breastfeeding.* Herb inhibits lactation; may worsen kidney disease or hypoglycemia.

NOTE: These precautions only apply to medicinal supplements. It is safe to occasionally eat foods that contain parsley.

OK Passionflower (*Passiflora incarnata*)

USE: Anxiety relief, sleep aid

STANDARD DOSE: 4 g to 8 g daily infused in tea

CAUTION: *Monitor infant for potential side effects.* If infant becomes excessively drowsy, stop taking the herb.

UNSAFE Peony Root (*Paeonia lactiflora*)

USE: Anti-inflammatory, for improved circulation, for treatment of polycystic ovarian syndrome

CAUTION: *Do not use if breastfeeding.* Herb inhibits lactation.

UNSAFE Peppermint (*Mentha piperita*)

USE: Anti-nausea, for treatment of IBS and indigestion

CAUTION: *Do not use if breastfeeding.* Herb inhibits lactation.

NOTE: These precautions apply to oral supplements or teas. When used appropriately, topical use of peppermint is not harmful and has anti-infective properties.

UNSAFE Pigeon Pea (*Cajanus cajan*)

USE: Anti-inflammatory, antidiabetic

CAUTION: *Do not use if breastfeeding.* Pigeon pea inhibits lactation.

OK Psyllium Seed (Blond) / Ispaghula (*Plantago ovata*)

USE: Laxative

STANDARD DOSE: 12 g to 40 g daily as powder in 5 oz of water or juice

CAUTION: Herb may take several days for laxative effects; may disrupt food absorption; may affect insulin dependent patients; may cause allergic reaction.

`UNSAFE` Pygeum Extract (*Prunus africanum*)

USE: For treatment of lower urinary tract infection

CAUTION: *Do not use if breastfeeding.* Pygeum inhibits lactation.

`UNSAFE` Rhubarb Root (*Rheum officinale, Rheum palmatum*)

USE: Laxative

CAUTION: *Do not use if breastfeeding.* May cause gastrointestinal distress (short term use) and/or electrolyte imbalance, albuminuria, hematuria, potassium deficiency and/or irregular heartbeats.

`UNSAFE` Rosemary (*Rosmarinus officinalis*)

USE: Anxiety relief, for memory and concentration, anti-infective

CAUTION: *Do not use if breastfeeding.* Herb inhibits lactation.

NOTE: These precautions only apply to medicinal supplements. It is safe to occasionally eat foods that contain rosemary.

`OK` Senna Leaf and Pod (*Senna alexandrina*)

USE: Laxative

STANDARD DOSE: 20 mg to 30 mg of hydroxyanthracene (active ingredient) infused in tea

CAUTION: *Monitor infant for potential side effects.* Senna is safe for breastfeeding as long as it is used on a 1 or 2 time basis, not at a high dose, and not regularly.

`OK` Siberian Ginseng (*Eleutherococcus senticosus*)

USE: For enhancing mental capacity, for fatigue

STANDARD DOSE: 2 g to 3 g daily as extract, or infused in tea, or in siberian ginseng soda, for up to 3 months

CAUTION: None for breastfeeding; use with caution in parents with hypertension.

`OK` Soy Lecithin (*Lecithinum ex soya*)

USE: For treatment of high cholesterol or recurrent plugged breast ducts

STANDARD DOSE: 3.5 g daily as liquid extract, granules, or capsules

CAUTION: None known

`OK` St. John's Wort (*Hypericum perforatum*)

USE: Anxiety relief, for mild depression, topical wound care

STANDARD DOSE: Orally, 300 mg (containing 0.3% hypericin) daily in the form of capsules, transdermal patches, or tea / Topically, as infused oil applied directly to minor wound several times per day

CAUTION: *Monitor infant for potential side effects.* When breastfeeding, monitor infant for abdominal symptoms (e.g., colic). Herb interacts with many drugs; do not use without consulting a doctor.

`UNSAFE` Uva Ursi Leaf / Bearberry (*Arctostaphylos uva-ursi*)

USE: Antimicrobial, for treatment of urinary tract infections

CAUTION: *Do not use if breastfeeding.* Possible disruption of formation of melanin (even while not breastfeeding, do not use for more than 7 days due to decreased formation of melanin).

`OK` Valerian Root (*Valeriana officinalis*)

USE: Anxiety relief, sleep aid

STANDARD DOSE: 2 g to 3 g daily taken in divided doses, in the form of capsules or infused in tea

CAUTION: *Monitor infant for potential side effects.* If infant becomes excessively drowsy, mother should stop taking the herb.

Recommended Alternatives to Unsafe Herbals

Note: Be sure to read additional information about the recommended alternatives in **Herbal Galactagogues** *(page 169) and* **Other Commonly Used Herbal Remedies and Products** *(page 175).*

TYPICAL USE	UNSAFE HERB	RECOMMENDED ALTERNATIVE
Major Galactagogues	*Anti-Galactagogues:* Barley Sprout Black Walnut Bugleweed Parsley Peppermint Sage	Blessed Thistle* Chasteberry / Vitex Fennel Seed* Fenugreek Seed* Garlic Goat's Rue Milk Thistle*
Minor Galactagogues	*Anti-Galactagogues:* Flannel Weed Osha Root Peony Root Pigeon Pea Pygeum Extract	Alfalfa* Anise Seed* Borage* Caraway Seed Coriander / Cilantro Seed* Dandelion* Dill Seed Fennel Seed* Hops Marshmallow Root* Oat Straw / Oat Tops Red Clover Red Raspberry Leaf* Stinging Nettle* Vervain
Analgesics	Comfrey	Bugleweed*
Anti-Inflammatory and Headache or Migraine Agents	Feverfew	Evening Primrose Oil*
Cough, Cold, and Allergy Products	Coltsfoot	Echinacea Elderflower
Anti-Asthmatic Preparations	Ephedra	No recommended alternative

Monitor infant for potential side effects

TYPICAL USE	UNSAFE HERB	RECOMMENDED ALTERNATIVE
Gastrointestinal Agents	Aloes Buckthorn Cascara Sagrada Bark Licorice Root Rhubarb Root	Chamomile Flower Flaxseed (Cracked) Psyllium Seed (Blond) / Ispaghula Senna*
Nausea and Vomiting Preparations	Peppermint	Ginger
Lipid Lowering Agents	Hawthorn	Soy Lecithin
Urinary Tract Infection Preparations	Butterbur / Petasites Root Uva Ursi Leaf / Bearberry	Cranberry* Goldenrod
Thrush Agents	Rosemary	Grapefruit Seed*
Anti-Anxiety Agents	Indian Snakeroot Kava Kava Root	Passionflower* St. John's Wort* Valerian Root*
Stimulants	Angelica Root / Dong Quai Ginseng Root	Ginkgo Leaf* Siberian Ginseng
Sleep Aid Preparations	Holy Basil Peppermint	Lemon Balm Melatonin
Antioxidants	Peppermint Rosemary Sage	Grape Seed*
Eye Health Products	Bilberry	Ginkgo Leaf* Grape Seed*

Monitor infant for potential side effects

7.
DIETARY PRODUCTS

Common Dietary Supplements

UNSAFE **Alpha Lipoic Acid**

USE: Coenzyme with antioxidant and antidiabetic properties

CAUTION: *Do not use if breastfeeding.* No information available for pediatric use or breastfeeding; caution is advised.

OK **Bromelain**

USE: Proteolytic enzymes used for anti-inflammatory, antitumor, and digestive properties

STANDARD DOSE: 500 mg to 2,000 mg daily in divided doses

CAUTION: *Monitor infant for potential side effects.* Scientific studies for safety during breastfeeding are not available; very large molecular size should greatly limit passage into breastmilk; pediatric doses exist; hypersensitivity possible; enzyme may increase heart rate at higher doses.

OK **Chondroitin Sulfate**

USE: For protective effects on cartilage

STANDARD DOSE: 800 mg to 1,200 mg daily in single or divided doses

CAUTION: None known. No pediatric concerns reported via breastmilk; very large molecular size should greatly limit passage into breastmilk.

OK **Coenzyme Q10**

USE: Antioxidant, cardiotonic

STANDARD DOSE: 150 mg to 600 mg daily in divided doses

CAUTION: *Monitor infant for potential side effects.* No pediatric concerns reported via breastmilk; large molecular size should limit passage into breastmilk; pediatric doses exist; hypersensitivity possible; avoid high doses.

CAUTION: *Read carefully before using*   187    **OK** *OK to use*   **UNSAFE** *Do not use*

OK **Glucosamine**

USE: For osteoarthritis

STANDARD DOSE: 1,500 mg daily in single or divided doses

CAUTION: *Monitor infant for potential side effects.* No pediatric concerns reported via breastmilk; supplement has low oral bioavailability; maternal plasma levels are almost undetectable; observe for gastrointestinal disturbances.

OK **Glutamine**

USE: For metabolic fuel, for digestive disorders

STANDARD DOSE: 7 g to 30 g daily in divided doses

CAUTION: *Monitor infant for potential side effects.* Scientific studies for safety during breastfeeding are not available; very large molecular size and maternal protein metabolism should limit passage into breastmilk; pediatric doses exist; observe for gastrointestinal disturbances.

OK **Immunizen Powder Capsules (arabinogalactan / colostrum / lactoferrin / yeast / beta-glucans)**

USE: For boosting immune system

STANDARD DOSE: 6 capsules with water 1 to 2 hours before meals for 10 days as needed

CAUTION: Product may cause gastrointestinal discomfort.

OK **Lysine**

USE: For recurrent herpes simplex infections

STANDARD DOSE: 1 g to 2 g daily in divided doses

CAUTION: None known. No pediatric concerns reported via breastmilk; maternal supplementation should not result in significant levels in breastmilk; pediatric doses exist.

OK **Melatonin**

USE: Sleep aid

STANDARD DOSE: 1 mg to 10 mg, in various oral forms of 0.5 mg to 5 mg, including extended release formulations, daily

CAUTION: *Breastfeeding parents should not take more than 3 mg daily*; mothers with autoimmune disorders, diabetes, and/or depression should avoid use.

OK Omega-3 Fatty Acids

USE: For cardiovascular health

STANDARD DOSE: Limit of 2 g daily from dietary supplements

CAUTION: None known. Safe at normal doses for use during breastfeeding.

OK Prebiotics

USE: For healthy gut bacteria, for digestive health

STANDARD DOSE: 4 g to 5 g daily

CAUTION: Abdominal discomfort, bloating, and gas may occur while your digestive system adjusts. If gas or bloating occurs, divide dose in half.

NOTE: Prebiotics are carbohydrates (mostly fibers) that humans cannot digest, but beneficial bacteria in the gut eat these fibers, resulting in better digestive health and fewer antibiotic-related health problems.

OK Probiotics

USE: Antidiarrheal, for supporting gastrointestinal colonization, for urinary tract infections, for vaginal candidiasis and bacterial vaginosis

STANDARD DOSE: Depends upon use (see product labels)

CAUTION: Observe for gastrointestinal disturbances; probiotic potential of lactobacilli found in breastmilk is similar to that of the strains commonly used in commercial probiotic products; pediatric doses exist.

OK Quercetin

USE: Antioxidant

STANDARD DOSE: 250 mg to 1,000 mg daily for up to 12 weeks

CAUTION: Observe for hypersensitivity. Neurotoxicity is the dose-limiting adverse effect; doses above 1,000 mg per day can cause nerve tingling and kidney damage.

UNSAFE SAMe

USE: Antidepressant, for pain disorders, for liver conditions

CAUTION: *Do not use if breastfeeding.* No data available for use while breast-feeding; more breastfeeding compatible preparations are available for these conditions.

Weight Management Products

The use of weight management products in nursing individuals is controversial. Diet and exercise provide a safe and effective alternative to drug therapy. This should be the preferred method for postpartum weight loss. Since it took nine months to gain weight during pregnancy, those who intend to lose weight should allow at least nine months relying on drug-free methods such as diet, exercise, and calorie burn-off from breastfeeding. Excessive postpartum weight loss can leave you feeling exhausted and run down, or can result in low breastmilk supply or lack of nutrients in breastmilk.

		SAFETY LEVEL (PAGE 19)
alli Weight Loss Aid Capsules *(orlistat)*	UNSAFE	L3
Applied Nutrition Green Tea Fat Burner Capsules *(caffeine / chromium / green tea extract / herbs)*	UNSAFE	L4
Applied Nutrition Green Tea Triple Fat Burner Liquid Soft-Gels *(bioflavanoids / caffeine / herbs / tea extracts / vitamins)*	UNSAFE	L4
Biotest Hot-Rox Extreme Capsules *(amino acids / caffeine / yohimbine)*	UNSAFE	L4
Carb Stopper Extreme Capsules *(chromium / herbs / vitamins / white kidney bean extract)*	UNSAFE	L4
Creatine supplement, generic *(creatine)*	OK	L3
Dexatrim Max Complex 7 Capsules *(caffeine / dehydroepiandrosterone / garcinia extract / herbs / minerals / tea extracts / vitamins)*	UNSAFE	L4
Exercise-enhancing supplement, generic *(beta-alanine / caffeine / citrulline)*	UNSAFE	L4
Hemp protein powders, generic *(hemp or mixed plant with hemp)*	UNSAFE	L4
HMB exercise-enhancing supplement, generic *(HMB)*	OK	L3
Metabolife Break Through Tablets *(caffeine / cayenne / green tea extract / L-tyrosine)*	UNSAFE	L4
Metabolife Extreme Energy Capsules *(green tea extract / herbs / magnesium / niacin / pantothenic acid)*	UNSAFE	L4
Metabolife Ultra Caplets *(caffeine / co-enzyme Q10 / garcinia extract / minerals)*	UNSAFE	L4

		SAFETY LEVEL (PAGE 19)
MHP TakeOff Hi-Energy Fat Burner Capsules *(green tea extract / herbs / L-tyrosine)*	UNSAFE	L4
Natrol Carb Intercept with Phase 2 Weight Management Capsules *(calcium / chromium / white kidney bean extract)*	OK	L2
Natural Balance Fat Magnet Capsules *(aloe / chitosan / malic acid / psyllium)*	UNSAFE	L4
Nature's Bounty Chromium Picolinate Extra Strength Tablets *(chromium)*	UNSAFE	L4
Nature's Bounty CLA Softgels *(linoleic acid)*	OK	L2
NOW CLA Nutritional Oil Softgels *(linoleic acid)*	OK	L2
NOW L-Carnitine Fitness Support Capsules *(L-carnitine)*	UNSAFE	L3
Prolab Enhanced CLA Tablets *(flaxseed oil / linoleic acid / safflower or sunflower oil)*	OK	L2
Protein powders, generic *(brown rice, casein, egg, mixed plant without hemp, pea, or whey)*	OK	L1
Stacker 2 Ephedra Free Fat Burner Capsules *(caffeine / green tea extract / herbs)*	UNSAFE	L4
Weight or mass gainer supplements, generic *(high carbohydrates / high proteins)*	OK	L1
Xtreme Lean Advanced Formula Ephedra Free Capsules *(amino acids / caffeine / calcium / flavones / herbs / vitamins)*	UNSAFE	L4
Zantrex Blue Capsules *(caffeine / herbs / niacin / rice flour / tea extracts / yerba mate)*	UNSAFE	L4

Artificial Sweeteners

Information Capsules:

 Concentrations of **ASPARTAME** (and **PHENYLALANINE**, a metabolite of aspartame) in breastmilk are generally undetectable. However, these products should be avoided if either of the breastfeeding pair is diagnosed with phenylketonuria.

 ACESULFAME POTASSIUM, **SACCHARIN**, **STEVIA EXTRACT**, and **SUCRALOSE** are also safe to take while breastfeeding, though there is less research available for saccharin and stevia extract.

Sweetener		SAFETY LEVEL (PAGE 19)	AVOID IF PARENT OR INFANT IS DIAGNOSED WITH PHENYLKETONURIA
Acesulfame potassium	OK	L1	
Aspartame	OK	L1	✽
Saccharin	OK	L3	
Sodium saccharin	OK	L3	
Stevia extract	OK	L3	
Sucralose	OK	L2	

Brand

Brand			
Equal *(aspartame)*	OK	L1	✽
Neotame *(acesulfame potassium)*	OK	L1	
NutraSweetM *(stevia extract)*	OK	L3	
Splenda Original *(sucralose)*	OK	L2	
Stevia in the Raw *(stevia extract)*	OK	L3	
SugarTwin *(sodium saccharin)*	OK	L3	
Sunett *(acesulfame potassium)*	OK	L1	
Sweet One *(acesulfame potassium)*	OK	L1	
Sweet'N Low *(saccharin)*	OK	L3	

OK *OK to use* UNSAFE *Do not use* 192 ✽ *Additional note applies*

Vitamins and Minerals

Vitamin and mineral supplements in low to moderate doses are generally safe for breastfeeding individuals to take, not exceeding the recommended daily value.

	100% DAILY VALUE		SAFETY LEVEL (PAGE 19)	DO NOT EXCEED 100% DAILY VALUE
Beta-carotene	3 mg	OK	L1	*
Biotin (B7)	300 mcg	OK	L1	*
Calcium	1000 mg	OK	L1	*
Chromium	120 mcg	OK	L1	*
Copper	2 mg	OK	L1	*
Folic acid (B9)	400 mcg	OK	L1	*
Iodine	150 mcg	OK	L1	*
Iron	18 mg	OK	L1	*
Magnesium	400 mg	OK	L1	*
Manganese	2 mg	OK	L1	*
Molybdenum	75 mcg	OK	L1	*
Niacin (B3)	20 mg	OK	L1	*
Pantothenic acid (B5)	10 mg	OK	L1	*
Phosphorus	1000 mg	OK	L1	*
Riboflavin (B2)	1.7 mg	OK	L1	*
Selenium	70 mcg	OK	L1	*
Thiamine (B1)	1.5 mg	OK	L1	*
Vitamin A	5,000 I.U.	OK	L1	*
Vitamin C	60 mg	OK	L1	*
Vitamin B6	2 mg	OK	L1	*
Vitamin B12	6 mcg	OK	L1	*
Vitamin D	400 I.U.	OK	L1	*
Vitamin E	30 I.U.	OK	L1	*
Vitamin K	80 mcg	OK	L1	*
Zinc	15 mg	OK	L1	*

* *Additional note applies*   193   OK *OK to use*   UNSAFE *Do not use*

8.
SOCIAL DRUGS

Caffeinated Drinks

An infant's ability to clear caffeine from their system is markedly reduced compared to adults, but caffeine ingested through breastmilk is usually insignificant if the breastfeeding parent's caffeine intake does not exceed a limited amount.

Less than 150 mg of caffeine, consumed two or three times a day, is the recommended limit for a breastfeeding parent. This would be equivalent to one or two cups per day of coffee, tea, or caffeine-containing soft drinks. Most energy drinks exceed the recommended amount of caffeine, so energy drinks should not be consumed.

However, if breastfeeding a newborn or premature newborn in particular, it is best to avoid caffeine altogether. If taking prescription **THEOPHYLLINE**-containing products, parents should also avoid drinks containing caffeine.

See page 154 for information about caffeine tablets. For the approximate caffeine content of popular beverages, see the tables below.

Coffee (8 oz cup / 236 mL)	CAFFEINE CONTENT (mg)
Cold brew	100
Decaffeinated	3–8
Drip method	176–240
French press	80–135
Instant	40–198
Instant decaffeinated	3
K-Cup	75–150
Percolated	102–124
Pour-over	80–185

Espresso Drinks	CAFFEINE CONTENT (mg)
Decaffeinated, single shot (1 oz / 30 mL)	5-10
Decaffeinated, double shot (2 oz / 60 mL)	10-20
Double shot (2 oz / 60 mL)	80–200
Ristretto shot (0.5 oz / 15 mL)	30–40
Single shot (1 oz / 30 mL)	40–100
Triple shot (3 oz / 90 mL)	140–300

Tea (8 oz cup / 237 mL)

Black, brewed	30–70
Black, decaffeinated, brewed	2–4
Green, brewed	20–50
Ready-to-drink, bottled	10–60

Soft Drinks / Soda (12 oz serving / 355 mL)

7-Up	0
A&W Cream Soda	29
A&W Root Beer	0
Aspen	36
Barq's Diet Root Beer	0
Barq's Root Beer	22
Big Red	38
Cherry Coca-Cola	34
Cherry Coca-Cola Zero Sugar	34
Coca-Cola	34
Coca-Cola Zero Sugar	34
Diet 7-Up	0
Diet Coke	46
Diet Dr Pepper	41
Diet Mountain Dew	54

	CAFFEINE CONTENT (mg)
Diet Pepsi	36
Diet RC Cola	36
Diet Rite	36
Diet Shasta Cherry Cola	44
Diet Shasta Cola	44
Diet Sprite	0
Diet Sunkist	42
Dr Pepper	40
Dr Pepper Cream	41
Fanta Orange	0
Fanta Orange Zero Sugar	0
Ginger Ale	0
Jolt	72
Kick	31
Mello Yello	53
Mountain Dew	54
Mr. Pibb	41
Pepsi	38
Pepsi Light	36
Pepsi Twist	38
Pepsi Zero Sugar	69
RC Cola	36
Shasta Cherry Cola	44
Shasta Cola	44
Sprite	0
Sugar-Free Dr. Pepper	40
Sugar-Free Mr. Pibb	59
Sunkist	41
Tab	47
Vanilla Coca-Cola	34

Energy Drinks (shot serving / 57 mL)

	CAFFEINE CONTENT (mg)
5-Hour Energy	200
Proper Wild	180

Energy Drinks (12 oz serving / 355 mL)

Red Bull	111

Energy Drinks (16 oz serving / 473 mL)

Bang	300
Monster Energy	160
NOS	260
Redline Xtreme	316
Reign Total Body Fuel	300
Rockstar	160
Spike Hardcore Energy	350

Energy Drinks (24 oz serving / 709 mL)

Rockstar	240

Alcohol

Yes, a breastfeeding mother can drink alcohol. One to two cocktails, glasses of wine, or bottles of beer usually result in insignificant levels of alcohol in breastmilk. This limited quantity is generally safe, though it depends on how fast the drinks are consumed, whether food is also consumed, how much the individual weighs, and how fast their body is able to break down the alcohol.

Exceeding one to two drinks per day can be extremely dangerous for your infant. Do not breastfeed while intoxicated. Chronic excessive drinking can result in breastfed infants experiencing mild sedation to deep sleep and/or hypoprothrombinemic bleeding. In general, heavy drinkers should not breastfeed.

Alcohol will leave breastmilk naturally as it is cleared from the body. The process will typically take two to three hours per drink, according to the CDC. ***If you have one drink, it is safest to wait at least two hours before breastfeeding. If you have two drinks, wait at least four hours before breastfeeding.***

If you consume more than two drinks, you do not have to "pump and dump," and doing so will NOT reduce the amount of alcohol in your breastmilk. You may pump and discard the breastmilk if necessary to relieve discomfort, but you will still need to wait an appropriate amount of time before breastfeeding.

If you drink at all, even just one to two drinks, the odor of alcohol may cause infants to consume significantly less milk than usual. Monitoring how much breastmilk your infant consumes is recommended.

Given a choice of alcoholic beverage, beer is preferable when breastfeeding. Beer contains barley and/or hops, which are galactagogues (ingredients that assist in breastmilk production). The rule of one to two drinks maximum per day still applies.

Nicotine

Cigarettes, low-nicotine cigarettes, vape pens, e-cigarettes, cigars, hookah tobacco, and all other tobacco-containing products are unsafe for breastfeeding parents to use, and can cause significant harm to infants. Exposing an infant to tobacco smoke (this includes second-hand exposure from any adult, in addition to exposure through breastmilk) dramatically increases the risk of Sudden Infant Death Syndrome.

Even smoking occasionally can expose your breastfed baby to nicotine and other toxic, cancer-causing ingredients. Nicotine and toxic byproducts are rapidly transferred into breastmilk, and it takes around ten hours for these ingredients to be cleared from breastmilk after just one cigarette.

Breastfeeding and smoking can reportedly cause vomiting, diarrhea, tachycardia (rapid heart rate), and restlessness in breastfed infants. Tobacco may also have a negative influence on breastmilk production and affect the energy requirements of breastfed infants.

If a mother is exposed to secondhand smoke, it has been shown to enter the milk supply in small amounts as well. However, if being exposed to secondhand smoke is unavoidable, it is not harmful enough to discontinue breastfeeding.

Nicotine patches also transfer nicotine to breastmilk, but without the extra toxic ingredients found in cigarette smoke. It is safe to continue breastfeeding while using nicotine patches, as long as the patches are not being used along with cigarette smoking. For more information on smoking cessation aids, see pages 54 and 153.

Marijuana (Cannabis)

The main psychoactive (mind-altering) chemical in marijuana is delta-9-tetrahydrocannabinol, or THC. Health effects of marijuana may include enhanced sensory perception, pain relief, and euphoria followed by drowsiness and relaxation, slowed reaction times, problems with balance and coordination, increased heart rate and appetite, problems with learning and memory, hallucinations, anxiety, panic attacks, psychosis, chronic cough, and frequent respiratory infections.

When using marijuana, THC passes from the mother's plasma into breastmilk. *Current evidence indicates that marijuana use during lactation may affect a breastfed infant's neurodevelopment, especially critical brain growth after birth*. Breastfed babies exposed to THC can have problems with feeding and development, both mentally and physically.

Edibles, while still containing dangerous THC and not recommended for breastfeeding mothers, are considered to be the best option for therapeutic use because they can be standardized by strength and dosage, whereas smoked marijuana cannot. Edibles also do not contain the heated byproducts in smoke that contribute to the toxicity. Exposure to marijuana smoke is at least as toxic as cigarette smoke, and may also increase the risk of Sudden Infant Death Syndrome.

Overall, when it comes to marijuana use, there is a great need for more empirical data based on scientific studies, followed by the process of careful labeling that all prescription and nonprescription drugs must undergo before being recommended for medical use. Thus, the use of marijuana in any form is controversial at best.

Under federal law (as of 2023), marijuana is an illegal Schedule I drug, meaning it has a high potential for abuse. Though many states have deemed it legal for medical and sometimes recreational use, U.S. courts have ruled that marijuana will remain federally illegal until legislation is passed to remove it from Schedule I status.

This is vitally important for parents to understand because Child Protective Services (CPS) defines illegal drug use based on the federal scheduling guidelines. *Parents in any state in the U.S. are liable to have their children taken by social services if they use marijuana for either medical or recreational purposes.* Damaging health effects aside, all parents should consider this information before using marijuana.

CBD (Cannabidiol)

Unlike marijuana, CBD is readily available across the country. It can be taken in the form of over-the-counter oils, lotions, sprays, gummies, drinks, pills, or capsules. In most states, these products do not have to meet the stricter laws regulating marijuana use.

"Full-spectrum" or "whole-plant" CBD products contain all of the compounds found in the cannabis plant, including a small amount of THC. Hemp-derived full-spectrum CBD products are supposed to contain less than 0.3 percent THC. These are federally legal, but may be illegal at the state level. It is currently unknown whether the low levels of THC in these products are negligible or still harmful when transferred through breastmilk. It is also possible for the amount of THC to be mislabeled since companies are not required to disclose the source/strain of their hemp, and there is little regulation in place.

There are some full-spectrum CBD products made specifically from marijuana plants that contain higher levels of THC. These are federally illegal and, with regard to breastfeeding, should be considered as dangerous as any other marijuana product.

On the other hand, CBD products labeled "broad-spectrum" or "isolate" are not supposed to contain any THC at all, and thus should not have any effects of THC use. That being said, there are probably very few of these CBD products that have been analyzed and assayed properly to determine whether or not they contain trace amounts of THC.

There is not enough research to know whether CBD alone, without THC, poses any risk to a breastfed infant. Until there are specific studies with data on CBD use during breastfeeding, it is not recommended.

Topical CBD products are less likely to transfer to breastmilk, though it is still possible for CBD to be absorbed into the bloodstream from lotions and creams applied to the skin. Breastfeeding individuals choosing to use CBD products do so at their own and their breastfed baby's risk.

APPENDICES

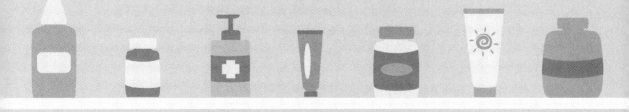

Appendix I: Helpful Words to Know

While reading this book you will come across a huge variety of product types and terminology. Please reference the following definitions for clarification.

Analgesic: A painkiller or pain reliever.

Anesthetic: A drug that causes temporary numbness or loss of sensation or awareness.

Antacid: A drug that neutralizes stomach acid.

Antibiotic: A drug that fights against bacterial infections by killing or preventing the growth of bacteria.

Antidiarrheal: A drug that relieves diarrhea or loose stools by slowing bowel movement and/or thickening stool contents.

Antiflatulent: A drug that relieves or prevents excessive intestinal gas.

Antihistamine: A drug that relieves or prevents allergy symptoms.

Anti-Infective: Any drug that treats or prevents infection, including antibiotics, antibacterials, antivirals, antiseptics, antifungals, and antiparasitics.

Antipyretic: A drug that prevents or reduces fever.

Antiseptic: A drug that reduces the likelihood of infection when applied to the skin.

Antitussive: A cough suppressant; relieves or reduces the urge to cough.

Astringent: A drug that causes body tissues to shrink and/or tighten, and dries up secretions such as skin oils or blood.

Contraindicated: A term used to describe a treatment that is not recommended due to conditions that may cause it to be harmful.

Corticosteroid: An anti-inflammatory drug that reduces swelling and inflammation; also called steroids.

Cosmetic: A product intended to have short-term, non-health-improving effects.

Decongestant: A drug that shrinks swelling in the nose to reduce sinus pressure and stuffiness.

Expectorant: A drug that breaks up mucus to help clear it from the lungs, throat, and sinuses.

Galactagogue: An herbal, food, or drug that is thought to help induce lactation or increase breastmilk production; also spelled *galactogogue*.

Gastrointestinal: A preparation or health problem affecting the digestive system, including the stomach and intestines.

H2-Receptor Antagonist: A type of drug that reduces stomach acid production, particularly for treating ulcers.

Herbal: A preparation that is made using plants. This can be in a variety of forms, including powders, tablets, extracts, juices, essential oils, teas, or simply dried or fresh herbs.

Homeopathic: An alternative medicine product intended to stimulate the body to heal itself with small doses of symptom-causing substances.

Intranasal: A preparation that is applied to the inside of the nose.

Lubricant: A drug that adds moisture and reduces friction or chafing.

Non-Steroidal Anti-Inflammatory Drug (NSAID): A type of drug that relieves pain and reduces inflammation and fever.

Ophthalmic: A preparation that is applied to the eyes.

Oral: Any preparation that is ingested via mouth, such as pills or tablets, or a preparation that is applied specifically to the mouth.

Otic: A preparation that is applied to the ears.

Preparation: A combination of active and inactive ingredients made ready for use. A preparation can refer to any form of medicine, including capsule, injection, liquid, suppository, suspension, tablet, etc. The term is often used for topical medications, but it is not exclusive to topicals.

Product: A specific preparation intended to relieve certain symptoms or have a certain effect on the user. A product includes a combination of active and inactive ingredients that is approved by the Food and Drug Administration (FDA).

Proton Pump Inhibitor: A type of drug that reduces stomach acid production, particularly for gastroesophageal reflux disease (GERD) or acid reflux.

Remedy: A product or other treatment used for a specific health concern.

Stimulant: A drug that increases activity in the body and nervous system, which can make a person feel more awake and energetic.

Sublingual: A preparation in the form of a tablet that is placed under the tongue, where it is dissolved and absorbed into the bloodstream.

Suppository: A preparation in the form of a small pellet inserted into the rectum or vagina, where it is either broken down to provide local symptom relief or is absorbed into the bloodstream.

Suspension: A preparation in liquid form, where the drug is not completely dissolved. It is important to shake suspensions before use to make sure the drug particles are evenly distributed in the liquid.

Therapeutic: A product that is intended to have long-term health-improving effects with continued use.

Topical: A preparation that is not ingested but rather applied onto a specific area of the body, such as skin cream or eye drops.

Treatment: Any medical care used for illness, injury, or other health concern.

Appendix II: Insect Repellent

Topical insect repellent, in the form of bug sprays, lotions, or wipes, can include ingredients such as DEET, picaridin, ethyl butylacetylaminopropionate (IR3535), 2-undecanone, citronella oil, oil of lemon eucalyptus, lemongrass oil, or peppermint oil. As long as the product is EPA registered or FDA approved, and is used in recommended doses with proper application, any amount of these ingredients present on the skin that would transfer to breastmilk would be negligible. Avoid getting product directly on the nipple area.

Repellents containing the insecticide permethrin are effective, particularly against ticks, but when used for this purpose, they should be applied to clothes or camping gear and not directly to your skin.

Appendix III: Treating Sore and Cracked Nipples

Sore, cracked nipples remain one of the top three reasons why parents stop breastfeeding. Up to 30 percent or more of mothers give up on the breastfeeding experience due to this problem, which then causes their babies to miss out on the powerful physical, emotional, and intellectual health benefits of breastmilk. With sore, cracked nipples, breastfeeding can be excruciatingly painful. With no sore, cracked nipples, the breastfeeding experience can and will be touchingly beautiful.

I have been counseling breastfeeding moms and their families for over four decades, doing my best to help every family maintain a positive breastfeeding experience for as long as possible. That is why I spent a decade developing a product to treat raw, sore, cracked, chafed, and painful nipples.

Various traditional treatments include application of expressed milk, warm water or tea bag compresses, heat, lanolin, vitamin A, collagenase, dexpanthenol, hydrogel or glycerin gel therapy, moist occlusive dressing, and education regarding proper latch and positioning. Naturally, education should be the first treatment. This includes learning to break latch and relatch, trying a different hold, and/or reclining while breastfeeding. A lactation consultant can help ensure that a baby is latching properly.

When proper latch and positioning are achieved, yet sore, cracked nipples persist, pharmacological treatments are the next step. However, products currently on the market are only marginally helpful.

Lanolin

The dominant form of treatment is lanolin ointment or cream. Lanolin (from Latin *lāna* 'wool', and *oleum* 'oil'), is a wax secreted by the sebaceous glands of wool-bearing animals. There are several issues concerning the use of lanolin for sore and cracked nipples:

- Can irritate sensitive skin and cause allergic reactions

- Does not provide protection against infection

- Chemically extracted from sheep's wool, leaving residual chemicals

- Non-breathable product, which can promote bacterial growth

Peppermint Gel

There are many other pharmacological products and methods on the list of possible treatments for sore, cracked nipples. One class of those products is hydrogels. The product I created, Dr. Nice's Moisturizing Gel, is part of that class of treatments. The peppermint gel's most unique property is its ability to turn into a cooling liquid when refrigerated. When applied, it once again becomes a soothing gel that fills in the cracks in the skin to form a breathable, protective layer preventing trans-epidermal water loss and infection. This product also contains peppermint oil in a safe and effective concentration.

In studies and reviews, peppermint has been shown to work both prophylactically (*prevents* sore, cracked nipples) and actively (*treats* sore, cracked nipples). Peppermint is an anti-infective, antibacterial, and antifungal.

If a mother ingests peppermint products in relatively high doses, it has the potential to decrease milk supply, but this effect has not been reported by any study or user of Dr. Nice's Moisturizing Gel to date. While breastfeeding, an infant is likely to ingest only about 0.00025 mL of peppermint oil (1/200,000[th] teaspoonful). For reference, a 1 oz serving of peppermint candy contains 0.4 mL to 0.8 mL of peppermint oil, which would be safe for children to eat.

Dr. Nice's Moisturizing Gel is the only water-based, vegan, all-natural product designed specifically for breastfeeding moms.

- FDA certified product
- Plant-based ingredients
- No parabens or petroleum
- FDA certified organic
- Cruelty free

Should you have any questions or comments about this product, please contact me through DrNiceProducts.com.

Appendix IV: Breastfeeding Medication Websites and Further Reading

DR. NICE PRODUCTS, LLC: https://www.drniceproducts.com

This website provides information about Dr. Nice's Moisturizing Gel product, as well as general counseling tips for pharmacists (www.drniceproducts.com/reference-materials), and further reading for parents (www.drniceproducts.com/blog). Healthcare professionals may contact Dr. Nice for consultation advice at no cost through the website.

INFANT RISK CENTER: https://www.infantrisk.com

The Infant Risk Center (IRC) is a worldwide call center presently in the Texas Tech University Health Sciences Center, School of Medicine, Department of Pediatrics in Amarillo and is directed by Dr. Thomas Hale. The Center is used by physicians, nurses, lactation consultants, and mothers in every part of the world. The IRC helps parents, lactation consultants, and doctors evaluate infant risk from exposure to multiple drugs, with the goal of continuing breastfeeding.

LACTMED SEARCH: https://www.ncbi.nlm.nih.gov/books/NBK501922/

Philip O. Anderson, a leading pharmacist and breastfeeding expert, originated LactMed as a peer-reviewed and fully referenced National Library of Medicine database of drugs to which breastfeeding mothers may be exposed. Maternal and infant levels of drugs, possible effects on breastfed infants and on lactation, and alternate drugs to consider can be found on this website.

BREASTFEEDING ONLINE: http://www.breastfeedingonline.com

Cindy Curtis, a registered nurse and International Board Certified Lactation Consultant developed Breastfeeding Online to help empower women to choose to breastfeed and to educate society of the importance and benefits of breastfeeding. She provides therapies for mastitis, thrush, engorgement, insufficient milk supply, and nipple vasospasm, among others.

NATURAL STANDARD DATABASE: https://pubmed.ncbi.nlm.nih.gov/20432139/

The Natural Standard Database contains systematic reviews of foods, functional foods, diets, supplements, vitamins, minerals, and Complementary and Alternative Medicine (CAM) modalities. It is designed to serve as a clinical decision support tool. This website will provide an overview of Natural Standard and its content and scope, as well as provide some basics for searching this resource.

AMERICAN ACADEMY OF PEDIATRICS POLICY STATEMENT: THE TRANSFER OF DRUGS AND OTHER CHEMICALS INTO HUMAN MILK: https://pediatrics. aappublications.org/content/108/3/776

The American Academy of Pediatrics places emphasis on increasing breastfeeding rates in the United States. A common reason for the cessation of breastfeeding is the use of medication by a nursing mother and advice by her physician to stop nursing. Such advice may not be warranted. This statement is intended to supply pediatricians, obstetricians, and family physicians with data, if known, concerning the excretion of drugs into human milk. Most drugs likely to be prescribed to a nursing individual should have no effect on milk supply or on infant well-being. This information is important not only to protect nursing infants from untoward effects of parental medications but also to allow effective pharmacologic treatment of breastfeeding parents. Nicotine, psychotropic drugs, and silicone implants are three important topics reviewed in this statement.

INDEX